Visual Aids to the MRCP Examination

To my wife, Olga,
and my daughter and son, Anita and Robin,
for their support and encouragement.

Visual Aids to the MRCP Examination

N.K. Chakravorty
MBBS, FRCP(E), DTM&H

Consultant Physician in Medicine for the Elderly
St Luke's Hospital
Crosland Moor
Huddersfield HD4 5RQ
UK

KLUWER ACADEMIC PUBLISHERS
DORDRECHT / BOSTON / LONDON

Distributors

for the United States and Canada: Kluwer Academic Publishers, PO Box 358, Accord Station, Hingham, MA 02018-0358, USA

for all other countries: Kluwer Academic Publishers Group, Distribution Center, PO Box 322, 3300 AH Dordrecht, The Netherlands

A catalogue record for this book is available from the British Library.

ISBN 0-7923-8873-9

Library of Congress Cataloging-in-Publication Data

Chakravorty, N. K.
    Visual aids to the MRCP examination / N.K. Chakravorty.
      p. cm.
    Includes bibliographical references and index.
    ISBN 0-7923-8873-9 (casebound)
    1. Internal medicine—Examinations, questions, etc. I. Title.
    [DNLM: 1. Medicine—examination questions. WB 18 C435v 1995]
  RC58.C45 1995
  616′.0076–dc20
  DNLM/DLC
  for Library of Congress   94-40907
                                                               CIP

Published in the United Kingdom by Kluwer Academic Publishers, PO Box 55, Lancaster.

Kluwer Academic Publishers BV incorporates the publishing programmes of D. Reidel, Martinus Nijhoff, Dr W. Junk and MTP Press.

Origination by Speedlith Photolitho Ltd., Manchester.

Printed and bound by Emirates Printing Press, Dubai.

Contents

Acknowledgements

I would like to acknowledge the following persons:

Mr Wilson (retired Consultant Ophthalmologist) for providing me with some illustrations and Mr Aggarwal (Consultant Ophthalmologist) for providing the illustrations and other necessary help.

Dr Evans (Consultant Radiologist) for assistance in interpreting some radiological illustrations.

My other colleagues in Huddersfield including the colleagues in Medicine for the Elderly.

Mrs S. Ellis and her colleagues in the department of Medical illustrations at The Huddersfield Royal Infirmary.

My son Robin (a dental surgeon) for helping me with the use of the computer and with some part of the manuscript.

Figure credits:

Figures 3, 13, 17, 53, 66, 71, 100, 129 are reproduced with permission from Bellamy, N. *Colour Atlas of Clinical Rheumatology*, Lancaster: MTP Press Ltd 1985.

Figures 10, 30, 55, 65 are reproduced from Frisch, B. and Bartl, R. *Atlas of Bone Marrow Pathology*, Dordrecht: Kluwer Academic Publishers, 1990.

Figures 14, 49, 79, 113, 132, 156 are reproduced from Salfelder, K. *Atlas of Parasitic Pathology*, Dordrecht: Kluwer Academic Publishers, 1992.

Figures 36, 44, 61, 80, 82, 93, 134, 153 are reproduced from Rowlands, D.J. *Clinical Electrocardiography*, London: Gower Medical Publishing, 1991, by kind permission of the author and ICI Pharmaceuticals.

Figures 27, 74, 143 are reproduced from Wight, D.G.D. *Atlas of Liver Pathology*, Dordrecht: Kluwer Academic Publishers, 1993.

Figures 31, 60, 114, 141, 149 reproduced from Bartl, R. and Frisch, B. *Biopsy of Bone in Internal Medicine: an Atlas and Sourcebook*, Dordrecht: Kluwer Academic Publishers, 1993.

Figures 62, 68, 87, 117, 137, 142, 148, 158 are reproduced from Verbov, J. *Essential Paediatric Dermatology*, Dordrecht: Clinical Press/Kluwer Academic Publishers, 1988.

Figures 15, 20, 45, 57, 138, 145, 146 are reproduced with permission of the authors from *Medicine International*, The Medicine Group (Journals) Ltd.

Figure 41 is reproduced with permission of Drs L. Taylor and R. W. Carslaw and the Wellcome Trust Tropical Medicine Resource.

Figure 52 is reproduced with permission of Professor P. J. Morris and *The Practitioner*.

Figures 85 and 155 are reproduced with permission of Professor E.A.M. Gale and *The Practitioner*.

Figures 2, 4 and 18 are reproduced with permission of *The Practitioner*.

Figures 96, 104 and 126 are reproduced with permission of *Geriatric Medicine*.

References:

Wyngaarden JB, Smith LH, editors. *Cecil's Textbook of Medicine*, 18th Edition. WB Saunders Company, 1988.

Edwards CRW, Bouchier IAD, editors. *Davidson's Principles and Practice of Medicine*, 16th Edition. Churchill Livingstone, 1991.

Introduction

A large number of doctors take the MRCP examination every year; unfortunately the highest percentage of failure occurs in the Part II examination, particularly in the clinical part. The candidates are expected to elicit the clinical features correctly and quickly; they are closely scrutinized by the examiners and therefore there is a certain amount of stress involved on the part of the candidates. In addition, they are also expected to identify features shown in the illustrations correctly and within the limited time, which causes additional stress. Therefore continued practice is the only way to improve clinical acumen and confidence to enhance the chance of success.

The book is designed for these candidates bearing in mind their particular requirements. Considerable information is gathered not only from the doctors who have already passed this examination but also from those who have been currently sitting the examination. The author has been taking part in teaching junior doctors for the last 22 years; most of his registrars passed the examination while working for him.

The book contains a large number of clinical photographs, X-rays (including CT scans), ECGs, haematology and histology slides which the candidates are likely to encounter in the examination. Every effort has been made to fulfil most of the requirements of the MRCP examination but at the same time the book has been kept to a reasonable size.

The answers to the questions are given at the back of the book and serve as a general and useful guide, but for detailed information it is suggested that referral be made to the appropriate books and journals.

Although the book is specifically designed for the MRCP candidates, it should also be helpful for candidates appearing in the PLAB test and other undergraduate and postgraduate medical examinations.

Question 1

This 65-year-old patient was admitted with respiratory tract infection.

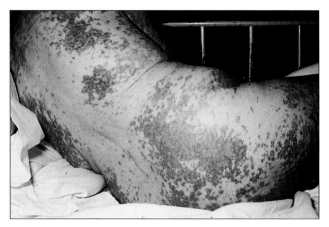

(a) What abnormality is observed in this patient?
(b) What is the likely cause?
(c) Name four other possible adverse effects which may result from the underlying cause.

Question 2

This 68-year-old female presented with deafness and deformity of the legs.

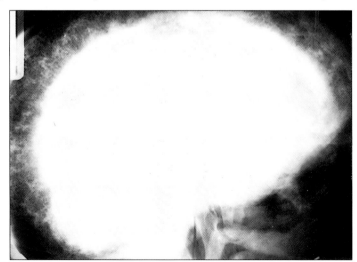

(a) What is the diagnosis?
(b) Name three useful investigations for this condition.

Question 3

(a) What does this show?
(b) What condition may it mimic?
(c) Name one investigation which may
    be helpful for diagnosis.

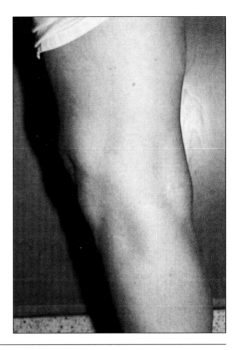

Question 4

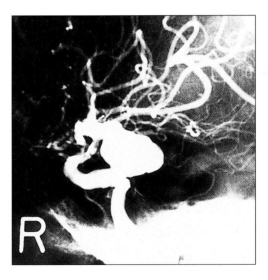

(a) What does this angiogram show?
(b) What complications may arise if it is not treated?
(c) Is angiography necessary and if so why?

Question 5

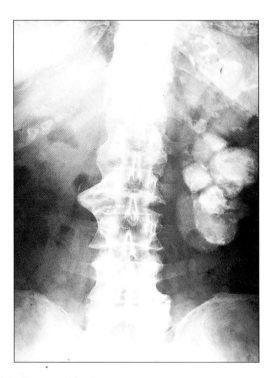

(a) What does this X-ray show?
(b) What was the underlying cause?
(c) What investigations would be necessary to diagnose the disease when it occurred?

Question 6

(a) What does the ECG opposite show?
(b) Name one underlying condition.
(c) What is the treatment?

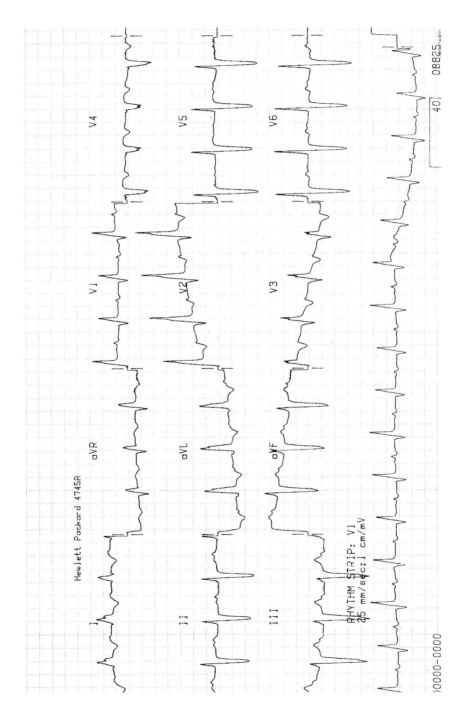

Question 7

(a) What does this X-ray of cervical spine show?
(b) What neurological complications may arise from this condition?

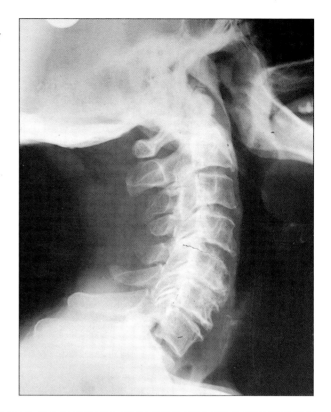

Question 8

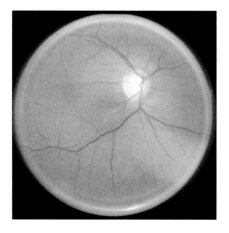

(a) What does this show?
(b) What are the underlying causes of this condition?

Question 9

(a) What does this X-ray show?
(b) Name three clinical features of this condition.
(c) Name two investigations to help the diagnosis; which one would you prefer and why?

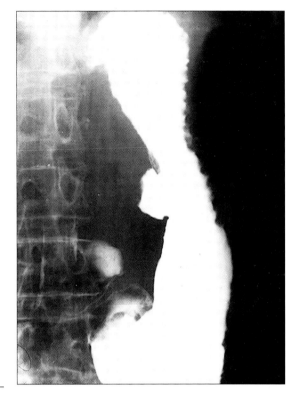

Question 10

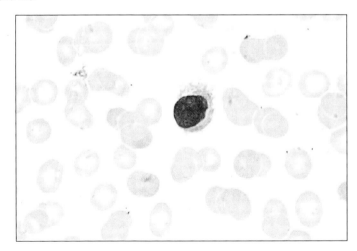

(a) What does this peripheral blood smear show?
(b) What are the features of this disease?

Question 11

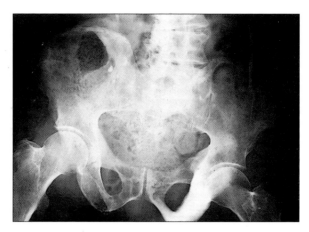

(a) What does this X-ray show?
(b) What may be the presenting symptoms of the patient?
(c) Name three other investigations you would like to carry out when the patient presents with the above symptoms.

Question 12

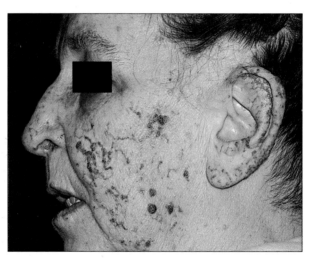

This 47-year-old patient presented with anaemia.
(a) What is the diagnosis?
(b) What is the inheritance?
(c) What is the most common presentation?

Question 13

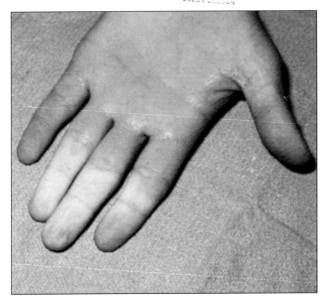

(a) What feature is shown here?
(b) What is the likely underlying cause?

Question 14

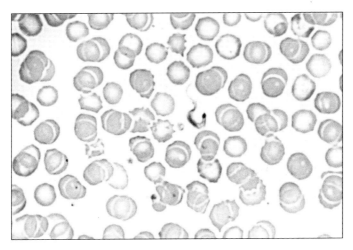

(a) What does this blood smear show?
(b) What disease does it cause?
(c) How is the disease transmitted to man?

Question 15

(a) What does this X-ray show?
(b) Name three features of this condition.
(c) What is the treatment?

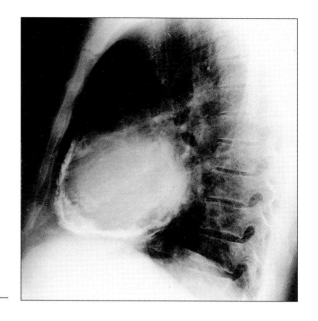

Question 16

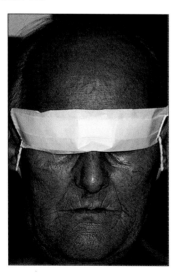 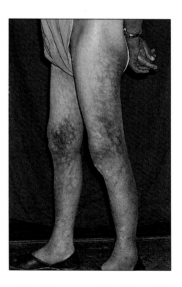

This fifty-year-old Caucasian male presented with generalized weakness and abdominal pain.
(a) What is the abnormality observed in this patient?
(b) What is the likely diagnosis?
(c) What is the inheritance?
(d) Name one investigation which will confirm the diagnosis.

Question 17

(a) What abnormality is shown on this X-ray?
(b) With what condition is this type of abnormality typically associated?

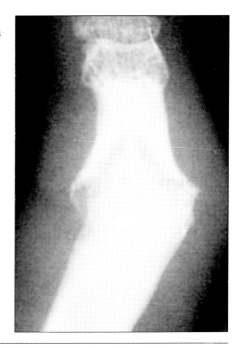

Question 18

This patient presented with a history of two epileptic fits.
(a) What is the abnormality seen on this CT scan?
(b) What is the likely diagnosis?
(c) What further investigation could be carried out?

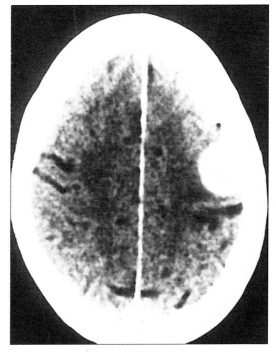

Question 19

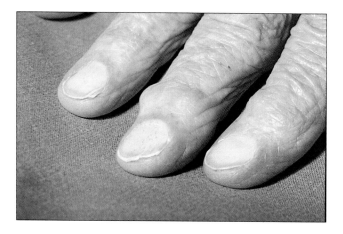

This patient presented with tiredness.
(a) What two abnormalities are seen?
(b) What is the likely cause of the abnormality of the nails?
(c) What may be the blood picture in this condition? (Name four.)

Question 20

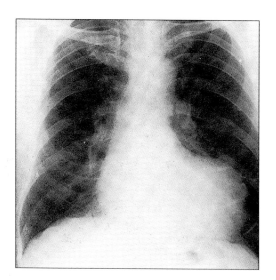

(a) What does this X-ray show?
(b) What is the diagnosis?
(c) What is the underlying cause?
(d) Name three possible complications of this.

Question 21

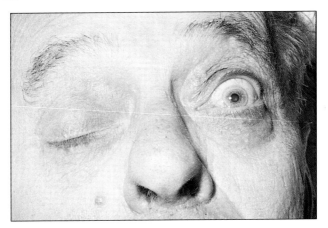

This 76-year-old patient presented with sudden onset of pain behind the right eye with inability to open the eye, following an argument with a neighbour.
(a) What is the lesion?
(b) What other examinations of the eye should be carried out to arrive at the diagnosis?
(c) What are the likely causes of this lesion?
(d) Name two useful investigations.

Question 22

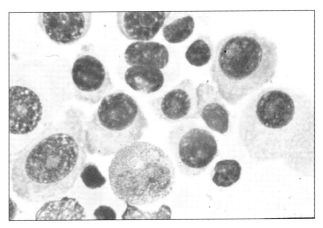

(a) What abnormalities are seen on this slide?
(b) What is the diagnosis?
(c) Name four important features of this disease.
(d) Name four other important investigations you would like to carry out in this disease.

Question 23

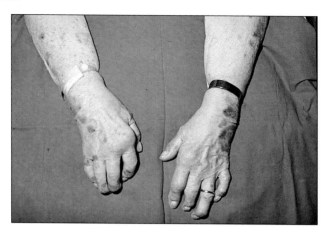

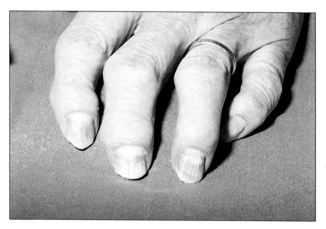

(a) What abnormalities are seen in this patient?
(b) What is the likely diagnosis?
(c) Name two investigations which will help the diagnosis.

Question 24

This patient presented with anaemia and haematuria.

(a) What does this abdominal CT scan show?
(b) Name two other features of this condition.
(c) Name three other helpful investigations.

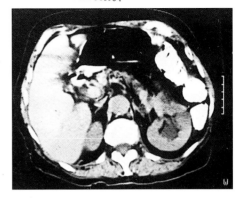

Question 25

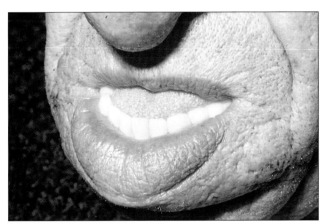

(a) What abnormalities are seen in this patient?
(b) What is the diagnosis?
(c) Name three other features of this condition.
(d) Name one investigation which will confirm the diagnosis.

Question 26

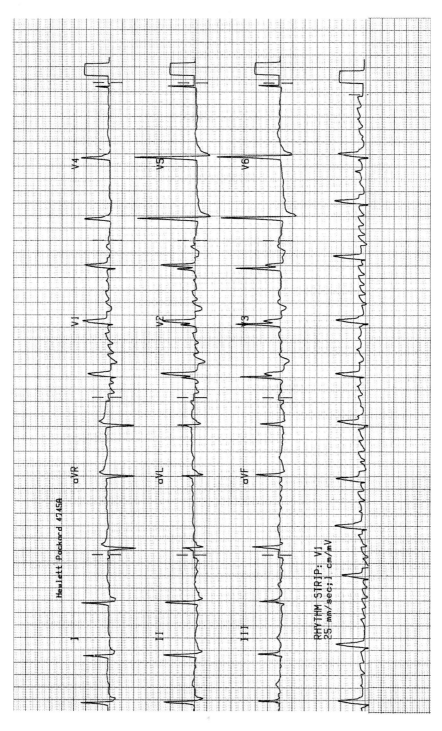

Question 26

(a) Name two abnormalities shown in the ECG opposite.
(b) Name two causes of each of the two abnormalities.

Question 27

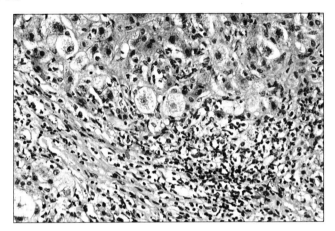

(a) What does this biopsy show?
(b) What is the likely diagnosis?

Question 28

This 75-year-old female presented with increasing swelling of the legs (non-pitting) and difficulty in walking.
(a) What is the likely diagnosis?
(b) Name two other conditions which may give rise to similar swelling.

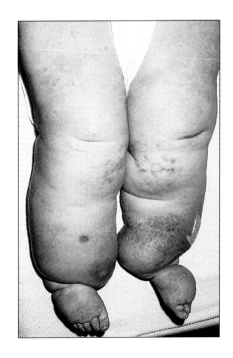

Question 29

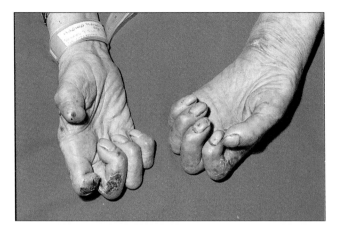

This patient complained of dropping objects while using her hands and difficulty in walking.
(a) List three abnormalities seen in this patient's hands?
(b) What is the diagnosis?
(c) Name five other clinical features which may be found in this condition.
(d) What other medical conditions could give rise to a similar picture?

Question 30

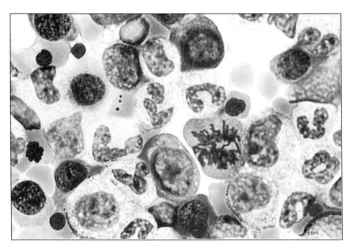

(a) What does this marrow show?
(b) What other diagnostic tests would you carry out?

Question 31

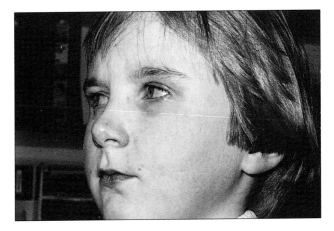

(a) What is the abnormality shown in this girl?
(b) What is the likely diagnosis?
(c) Name another important feature of the condition.

Question 32

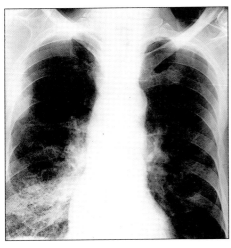 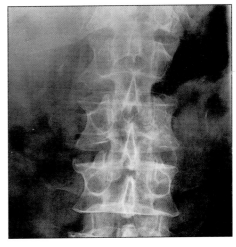

(i)   (ii)

This patient with a history of long-standing chronic obstructive airways disease presented with cough and yellowish expectoration, right-sided chest pain and severe backache.
(a) What do X-rays (i) and (ii) show?
(b) What are the diagnoses?

Question 33

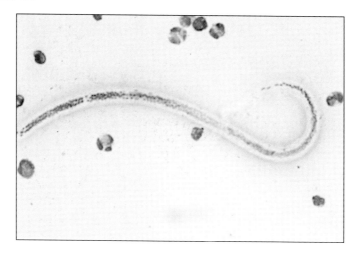

(a) What does this blood smear show?
(b) How is it conveyed to man?
(c) Name common features of this disease.

Question 34

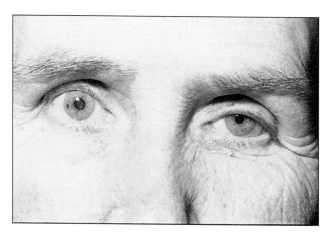

(a) What condition do the clinical appearances suggest?
(b) What are the characteristic features of this condition?
(c) Name three medical conditions which may give rise to these features.

Question 35

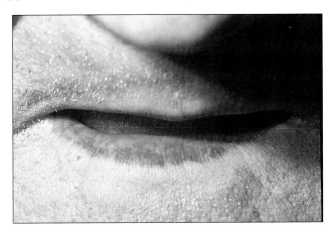

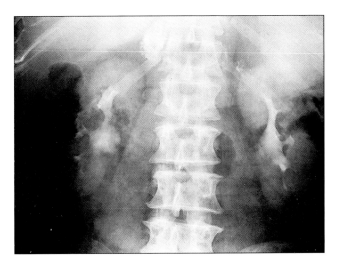

This patient presented with tiredness and dizziness.
(a) Name two abnormalities seen in this patient.
(b) What is the likely diagnosis?
(c) Name three aetiological conditions of this disease.
(d) Name three other features of this condition.

Question 36

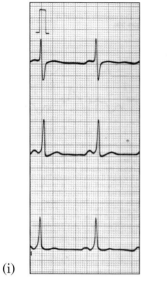

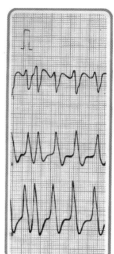

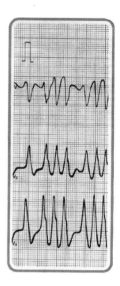

(i)   (ii)

(a) What do ECGs (i) and (ii) show?
(b) What is the cause?
(c) What may be the risk to the patients?
(d) What drugs may be used to treat this condition?

Question 37

This patient presented with acute onset of pain in the foot.
(a) What abnormalities are seen in this foot?
(b) What is the diagnosis?
(c) What is the usual mode of onset?
(d) Name three drugs which are used to treat this condition.

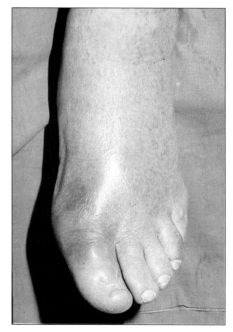

Question 38

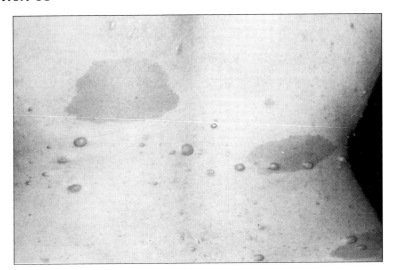

(a) Name two abnormalities seen in this patient.
(b) What is the diagnosis?
(c) What is the inheritance?
(d) Name three disorders associated with this condition.

Question 39

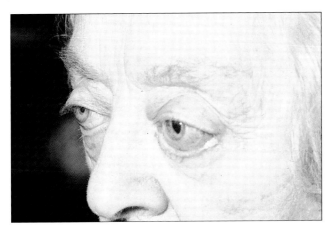

(a) What abnormality is seen in this patient?
(b) Name three conditions which can give rise to this abnormality.

Question 40

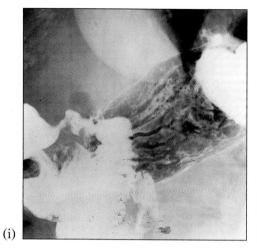
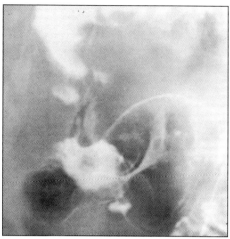

(i)　　　　　　　　　　　　　　　　　　　　　　　　　　(ii)

(a) What do X-rays (i) and (ii) show?
(b) How will you investigate the patient?
(c) Name two drugs which are used to treat this condition.

Question 41

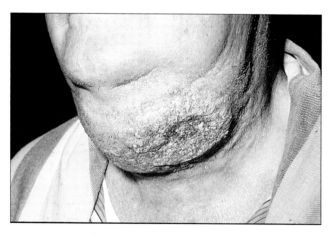

(a) What is this lesion?
(b) How is it contracted by humans?
(c) Name two possible serious complications.
(d) What is the treatment?

Question 42

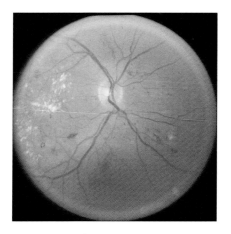

(a) What does this fundus show?
(b) Name four other clinical features of this condition.

Question 43

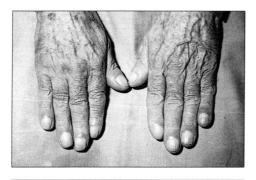

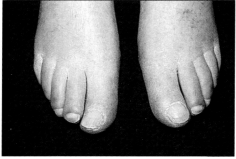

(a) What abnormalities are seen in this patient?
(b) What changes are responsible for this condition?
(c) Name four diseases which may give rise to this abnormality.

Question 44

(a) What does this ECG show?
(b) Does it indicate an organic heart disease?
(c) Is there any other abnormality that the patient is likely to have?

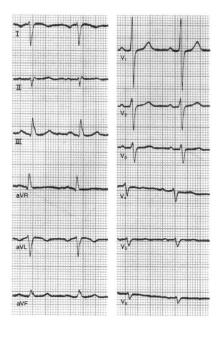

Question 45

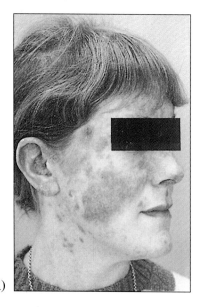

(i)

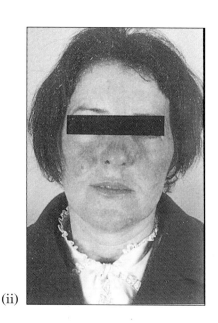

(ii)

(a) What abnormalities are seen?
(b) Name three other common features of this disease.
(c) Name the one most useful diagnostic laboratory finding.

Question 46

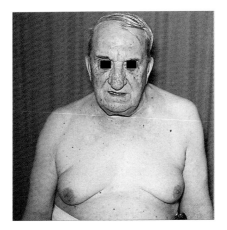

This seventy-year-old patient was treated for long-standing congestive cardiac failure.
(a) What is this abnormality?
(b) Name five underlying causes.

Question 47

This 70-year-old patient had an illness of prolonged backache and fever when he was young.
(a) What is the feature?
(b) What was the underlying cause of this condition?
(c) How common is this disease now in the Western world?

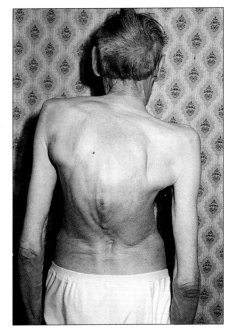

Question 48

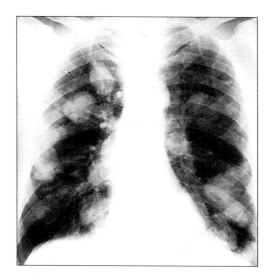

(a) What does this chest X-ray show?
(b) What are the likely primary lesions?

Question 49

(a) What does this X-ray show?
(b) Name four features of this condition.
(c) How would you diagnose it?

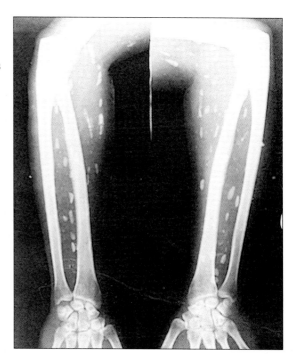

Question 50

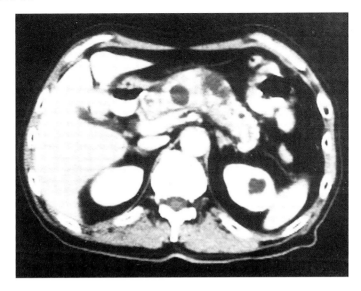

(a) Name two abnormalities shown on this abdominal CT scan.
(b) Name three clinical features of this condition.
(c) Name four other investigations for this condition.

Question 51

(a) What is the abnormality shown in the legs?
(b) Why does it occur?
(c) Which patients are prone to develop this condition?

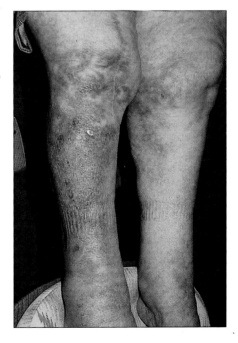

Question 52

(a) What does this angiogram show?
(b) Name four features of this condition.
(c) Which patients are likely to benefit from surgery?

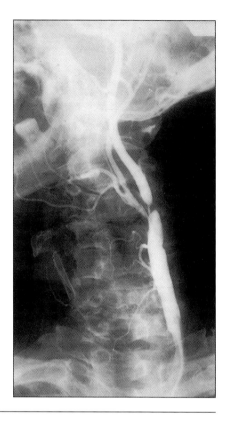

Question 53

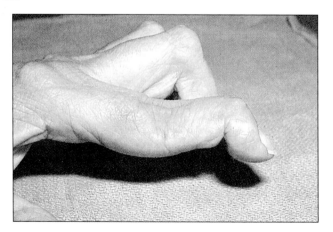

(a) What is the abnormality?
(b) Name three common clinical features at the onset of the disease.
(c) Name four extra-articular manifestations of this disease.

Question 54

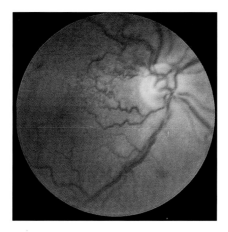

(a) What does this show?
(b) What effect might this have on visual acuity at various stages of the underlying disease?

Question 55

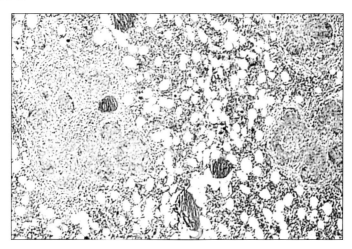

(a) What does this bone biopsy show?
(b) What radiological investigations may be helpful in this condition?

Question 56

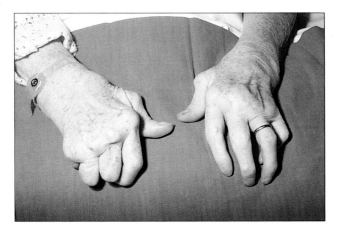

(a) What abnormalities are seen in these hands?
(b) What is the diagnosis?

Question 57

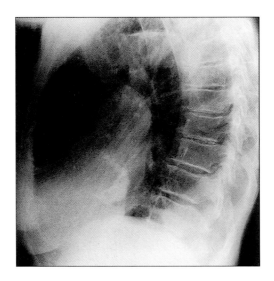

(a) What does this lateral view chest X-ray show?
(b) What can it be confused with?
(c) Name two conditions which may be associated with this.

Question 58

This patient presented with
increasing confusion.
(a) What does this CT scan
    show?
(b) What is the likely diagnosis?
(c) Name four key features of
    this condition.
(d) Name three other
    investigations which should
    be carried out to exclude any
    underlying causes.

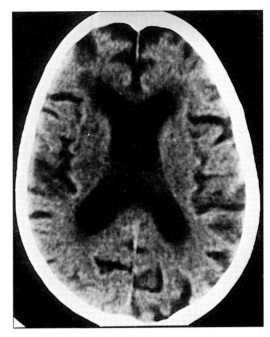

Question 59

(a) What are the abnormalities seen in
    this hand?
(b) What is the diagnosis?
(c) What are the likely initial
    symptoms?

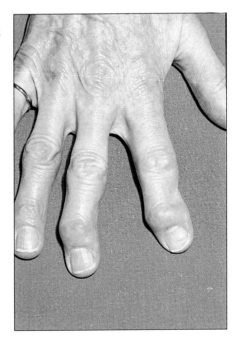

Question 60

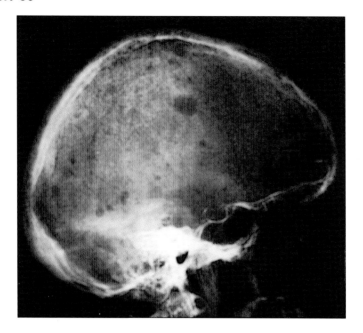

(a) What does this X-ray show?
(b) What is the likely diagnosis?
(c) Name four other features of this condition.

Question 61

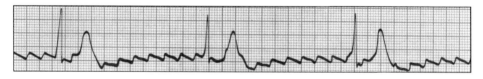

(a) What does lead III of this ECG show?
(b) Is it a common combination?

Question 62

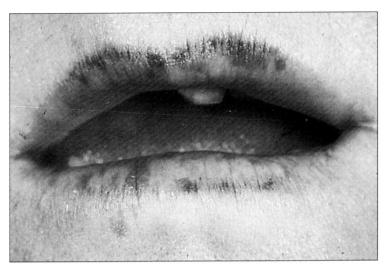

(a) What abnormality is shown in this patient?
(b) What other abnormality is associated with this condition?

Question 63

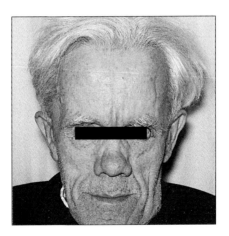

(a) What is the abnormality seen in this patient?
(b) Name three other features of this condition.
(c) Name three drugs used to treat this condition.

Question 64

(a) What does this X-ray show?
(b) Name two biochemical investigations which will help the diagnosis.
(c) Name three other radiological findings which may be present in this condition.

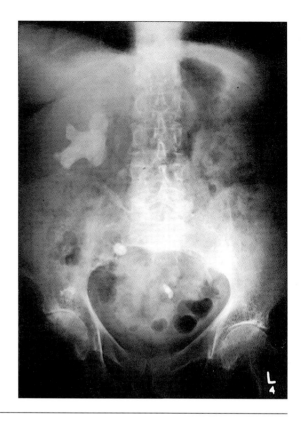

Question 65

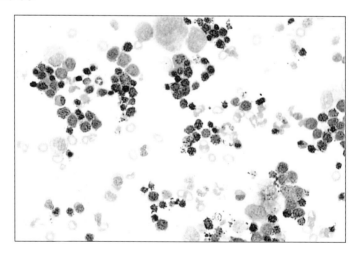

(a) What does this bone marrow aspirate show?
(b) How is the disease classified?

Question 66

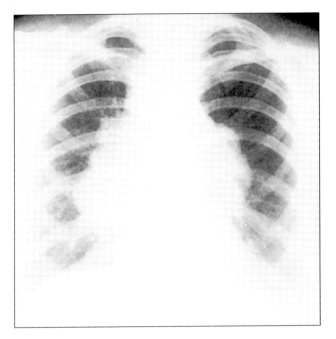

(a) What does this X-ray show?

(b) Name two possible underlying causes.

Question 67

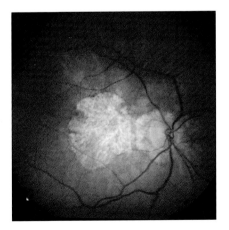

(a) What does this show?

(b) What effect does this have on the patient?

Question 68

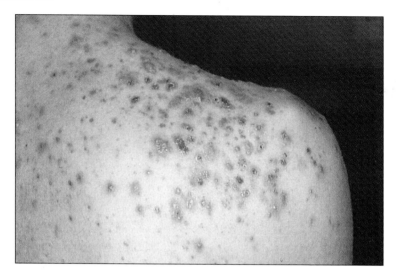

(a) What is this lesion?
(b) What is the common age for this condition?
(c) What treatment should be recommended?

Question 69

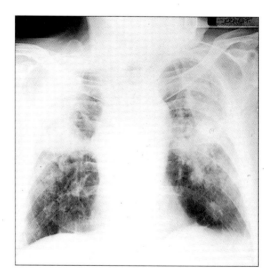

(a) What does this X-ray show?
(b) What is the likely complication of this condition?

Question 70

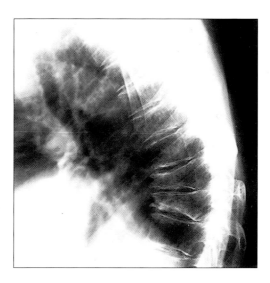

(a) What does this X-ray show?
(b) What are the clinical features?
(c) Name three other investigations which may be helpful in the diagnosis.

Question 71

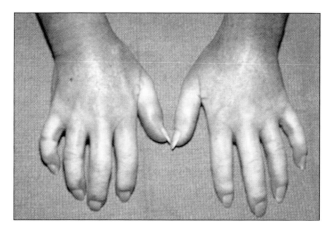

(a) What abnormalities are seen in the hands?
(b) What is the diagnosis?
(c) Name two other features of this condition.

Question 72

(a) What does this X-ray show?
(b) What are the likely causes?
(c) What is the symptom the patient is most likely to have?
(d) What other investigations should be carried out?

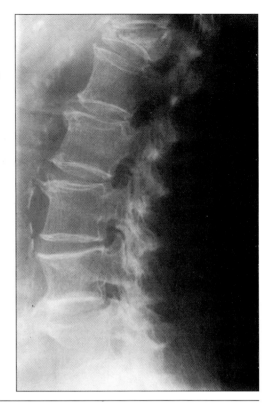

Question 73

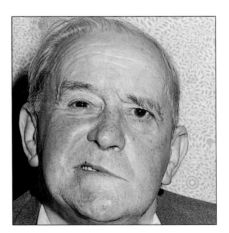

(a) What is the abnormality seen in this patient?
(b) What is the likely diagnosis?
(c) Where is the lesion?
(d) Name two other conditions which may resemble this.

Question 74

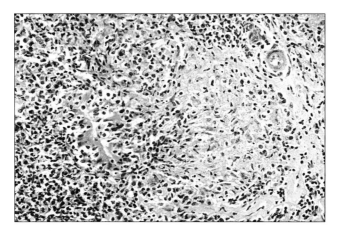

This 45-year-old female presented with pruritus and jaundice.
(a) What does this biopsy show?
(b) What is the likely diagnosis?
(c) Name three other features of this condition.

Question 75

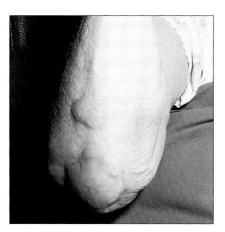

(a) What are the lesions?
(b) What is the significance of this?
(c) Name three other common sites of this lesion.
(d) What is the histological appearance?

Question 76

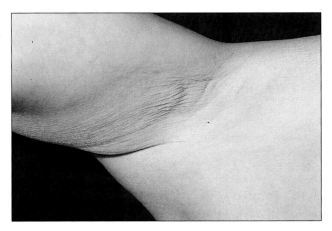

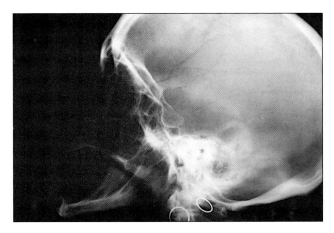

This male patient had decreased frequency of shaving (once a week) and had impotence.
(a) What abnormalities are seen?
(b) What is the likely underlying cause?
(c) Name three other features of this condition.

Question 77

This patient presented with increasing difficulty in walking and had evidence of bilateral pyramidal tract lesion.

(a) What does this X-ray show?
(b) Name two likely causes.
(c) What is the alternative non-invasive investigation which can give even more satisfactory information?

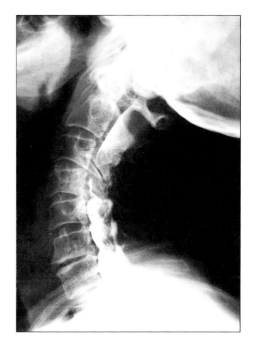

Question 78

(a) What abnormality do you see in this patient?
(b) What may be the underlying causes (name three)?
(c) How will you investigate this patient?

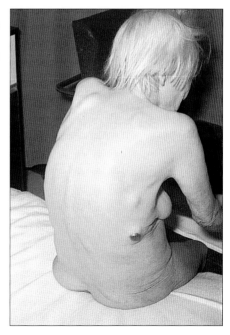

Question 79

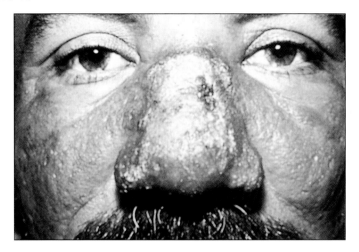

(a) What is this lesion?
(b) What is the causative agent of this lesion?
(c) What are the reservoir hosts and vectors of this parasite?

Question 80

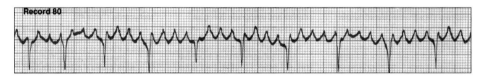

(a) What does this ECG show?
(b) Can it be difficult to distinguish from some other similar conditions and if so, what test may clarify the situation?

Question 81

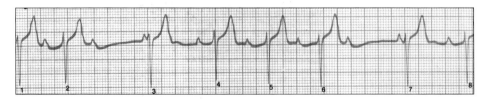

(a) What does this ECG show?
(b) What is this due to?

Question 82

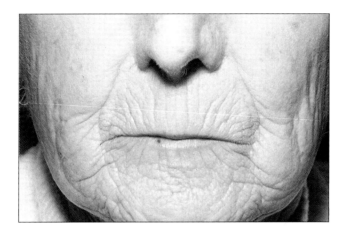

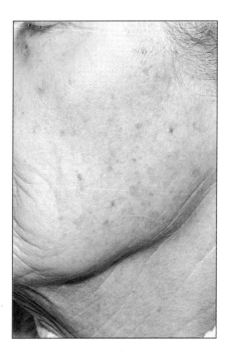

(a) What abnormalities are seen?
(b) What is the diagnosis?
(c) What is the most common mode of onset of this condition?

Question 83

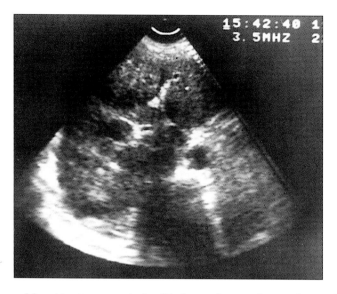

This 70-year-old patient presented with loss of appetite and weight.
(a) What does this abdominal ultrasound show?
(b) Name three underlying causes.

Question 84

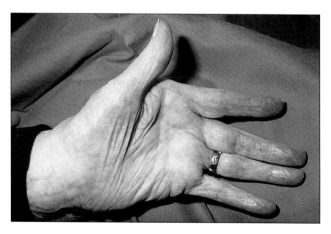

(a) Name two abnormalities seen in this hand.
(b) What is the underlying disease?

Question 85

(a) What is the abnormality seen in this young man, which he noticed following a minor injury (as a coincidence)?
(b) What is the underlying disease?
(c) Name two other conditions which can give rise to this.

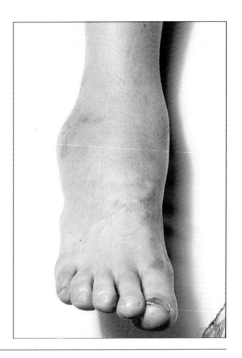

Question 86

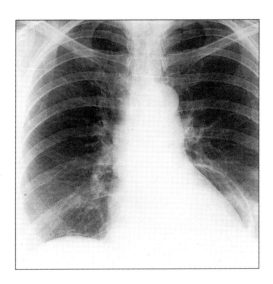

(a) What does this X-ray show?
(b) Name three features of this condition.
(c) What two investigations may be carried out?

Question 87

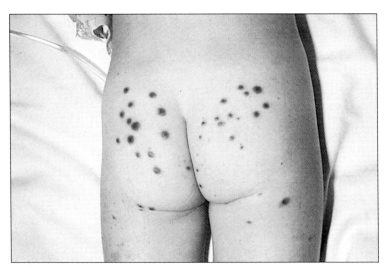

(a) What is this lesion?
(b) What is the cause?
(c) Name four associated features of this condition.

Question 88

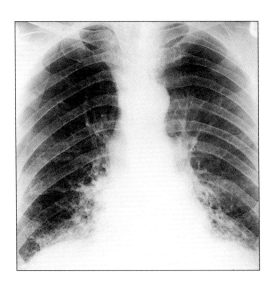

(a) What does this X-ray show?
(b) What is the likely diagnosis?
(c) Name three features of this condition.
(d) How can the diagnosis be made with certainty?

Question 89

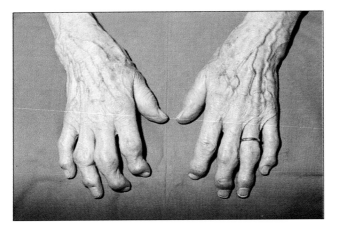

(a) What are the abnormalities?
(b) What is the diagnosis?

Question 90

(a) What is this condition?
(b) What is the cause?
(c) Name three possible sequelae.
(d) What is the preferred treatment?

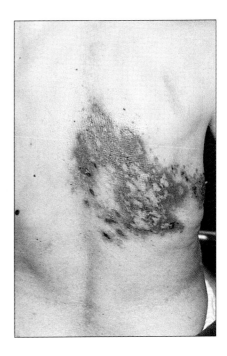

Question 91

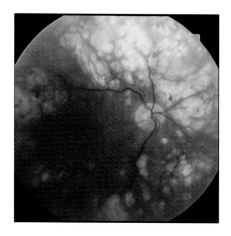

(a) What are the features?
(b) What complications may arise if this condition is not treated early?

Question 92

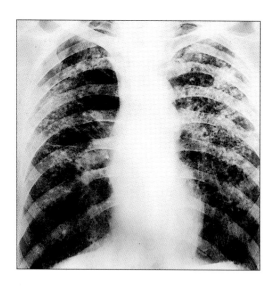

(a) What does this X-ray show?
(b) Name two underlying conditions.

Question 93

(a) What does the ECG opposite show?
(b) What may be the underlying cause?

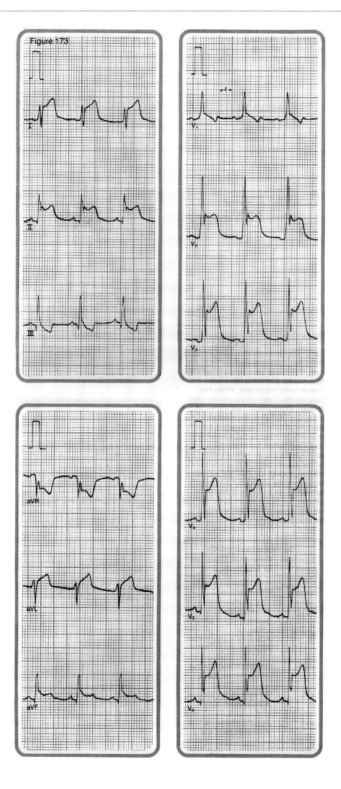

Figure 173

Question 94

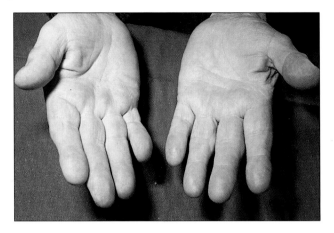

(a) What abnormalities do you see in these hands?
(b) What is the likely diagnosis?
(c) Name four other causes of similar abnormalities.

Question 95

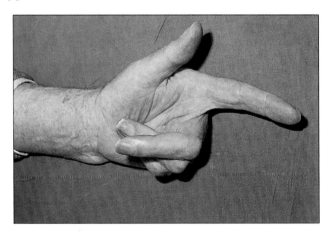

(a) What abnormality do you see in this hand?
(b) How is the deformity caused?
(c) Name three possible predisposing factors responsible for this condition.
(d) Is there a sex predilection for this condition?

Question 96

This patient presented with difficulty in walking.
(a) Name two abnormalities seen.
(b) What is the likely underlying cause?
(c) Name two investigations which will help diagnosis.

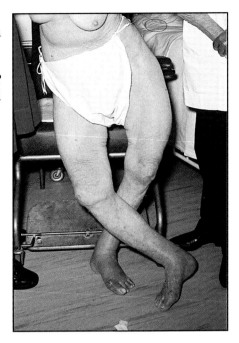

Question 97

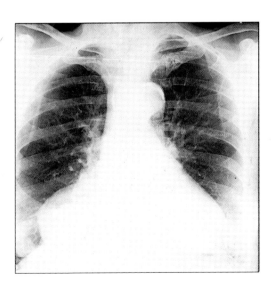

(a) What does this X-ray show?
(b) Does it require further investigations?
(c) What are the other likely causes?

Question 98

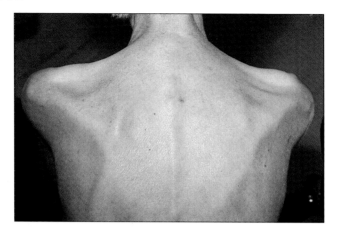

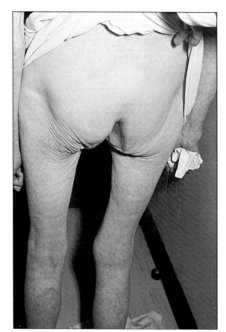

This patient presented with loss of weight but normal appetite.
(a) What abnormality is seen in this patient?
(b) What is the underlying disease?
(c) Name three other features of the disease.
(d) What investigations would confirm the diagnosis?

Question 99

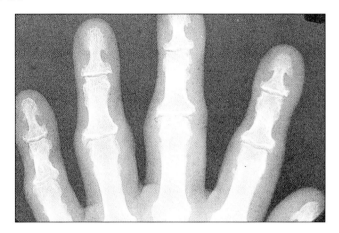

(a) What does this X-ray show?
(b) What other feature of hand X-rays is likely to help the diagnosis?

Question 100

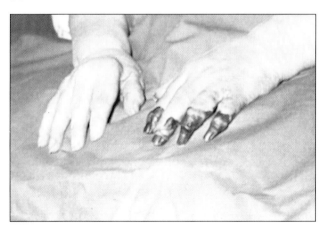

(a) What does this show?
(b) What is the likely underlying cause?

Question 101

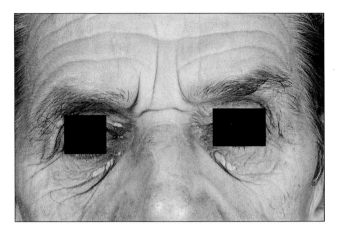

(a) What abnormality is seen in this patient?
(b) What is the likely underlying disorder?
(c) What condition may be associated with this abnormality?

Question 102

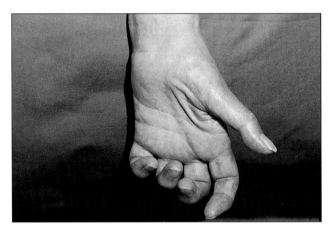

This patient presented with weakness of muscles of limbs and fasciculation but had no intellectual impairment or sensory deficits.
(a) What is the abnormality?
(b) What is the most likely diagnosis?

Question 103

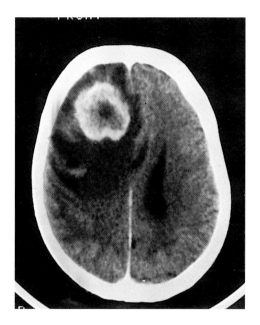

An elderly female presented with confusion; she was a heavy smoker.
(a) What does this CT scan show?
(b) What other radiological examination is likely to be helpful for the diagnosis?

Question 104

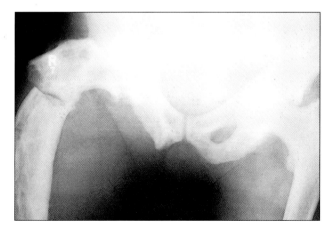

(a) Name three abnormalities seen on this X-ray.
(b) Name three possible complications of this disease.
(c) What is the incidence of this disease?

Question 105

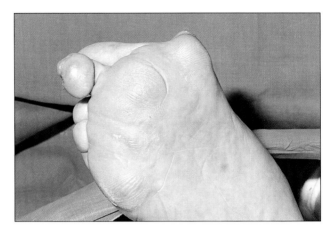

This patient, with a chronic inflammatory polyarthritis, complained of pain in the foot.
(a) What is the abnormality seen?
(b) What is the most likely underlying disease?

Question 106

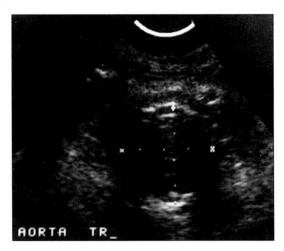

This patient was referred to the outpatient department with chest symptoms (cough and breathlessness). Routine clinical examination revealed an abdominal mass.
(a) What does this ultrasound show?
(b) Is there a sex predilection for this condition?
(c) What is the risk of this condition if not treated?

Question 107

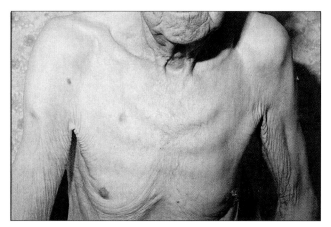

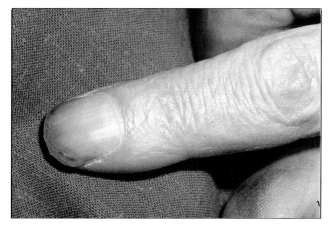

This patient presented with cough and loss of weight.
(a) What abnormalities are seen?
(b) What may be the likely cause?
(c) Name three investigations which will help the diagnosis.

Question 108

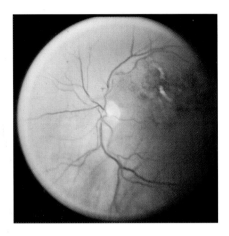

(a) What does this fundus show?
(b) What other condition should it be distinguished from?
(c) What effect does it have on the patient?

Question 109

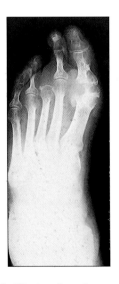 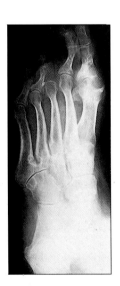

(a) What does this X-ray show?
(b) What is the diagnosis?

Question 110

(a) What are the abnormalities seen?
(b) What is the likely diagnosis?
(c) Name three other features of this disease.
(d) Name two investigations to establish the diagnosis.

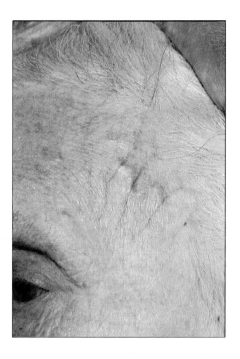

Question 111

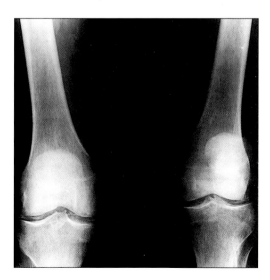

This elderly patient presented with acute pain in the knee joints.
(a) What abnormality is seen on this X-ray?
(b) How can the diagnosis be made?

Question 112

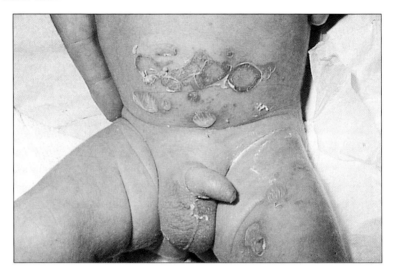

(a) What skin abnormality is shown in this two-week-old baby?
(b) Name two organisms which may be responsible for this.

Question 113

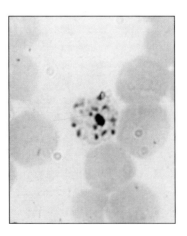

(a) What does this show?
(b) Name three features of illness caused by this.

Question 114

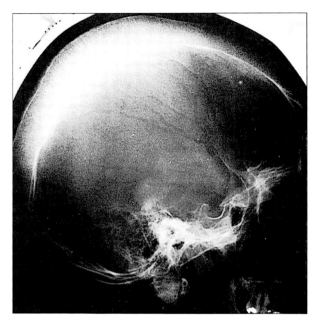

(a) What does this X-ray of the skull of a child show?
(b) What is the likely diagnosis?
(c) Name three other features of this condition.

Question 115

This patient presented with generalized weakness and confusion.
(a) Name two features seen.
(b) What is the likely diagnosis?
(c) Name five investigations which will help the diagnosis.

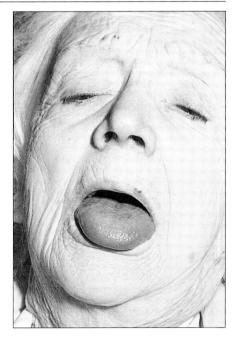

Question 116

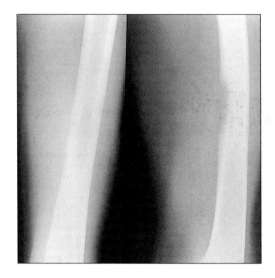

(a) What is the abnormality seen on this X-ray?
(b) What are the likely underlying causes?

Question 117

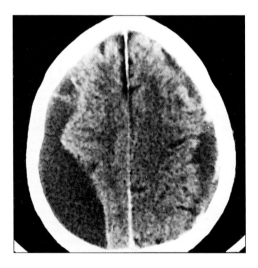

This elderly epileptic patient was admitted to hospital with drowsiness following a fall.
(a) What does this CT scan show?
(b) Which patients are prone to this condition?
(c) Name five features which may be present in this condition.

Question 118

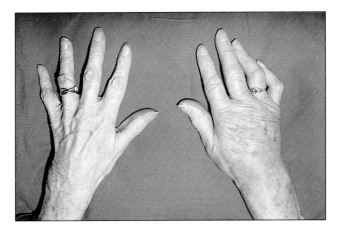

This patient developed a sudden pain and swelling of the dorsum of one hand. The problem disappeared in about a week following treatment with indomethacin.
(a) What is the likely diagnosis?
(b) Name one investigation which may help diagnosis.

Question 119

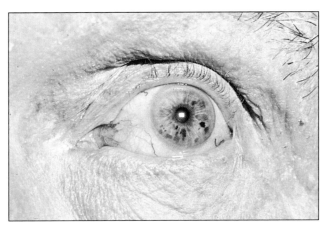

(a) What is the abnormality?
(b) What are the likely causes (name three)?
(c) Name two investigations which may be helpful in diagnosis.

Question 120

This patient presented
with difficulty in walking.
(a) What abnormality is
    seen?
(b) What is the likely
    cause?
(c) What other features of
    this disease may be
    seen in a child?
(d) What other
    investigations should
    be carried out in a child
    presenting with this
    problem?

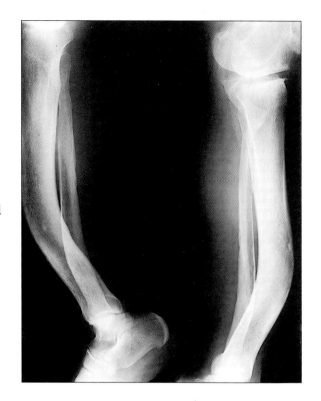

Question 121

This patient presented with frequent
falls.
(a) What is the diagnosis?
(b) Name three features of this
    condition.
(c) Name three drugs used to treat this
    condition.

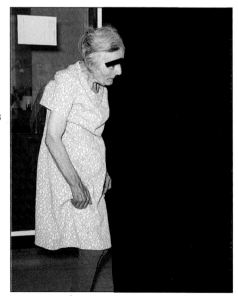

Question 122

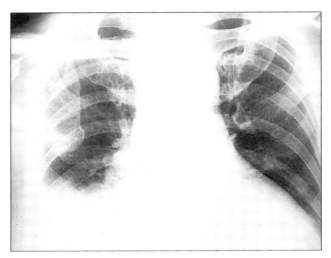

(a) What does this chest X-ray show?
(b) Name four other investigations which are likely to be helpful in determining the underlying cause of this condition.

Question 123

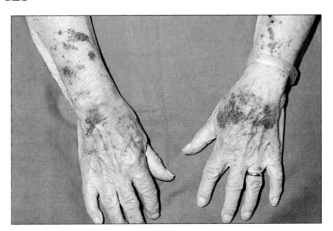

(a) What feature is seen?
(b) What is this condition?
(c) What is the pathology?

Question 124

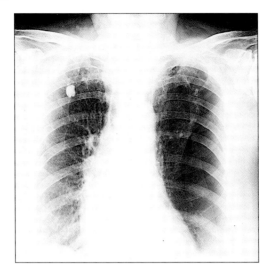

This patient presented with chest pain and breathlessness.
(a) What is the abnormality?
(b) Name two causes giving rise to this condition.
(c) Name three other features of this condition.

Question 125

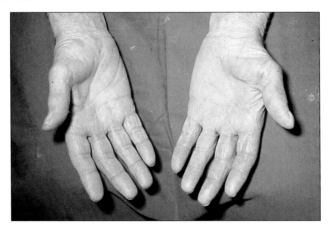

(a) What feature is seen?
(b) What is the likely diagnosis?
(c) Name two other clinical features of this condition.
(d) Name four possible underlying causes.

Question 126

(a) What is the deformity?
(b) What is the likely cause?
(c) Is hypercalcaemia usually found in this condition?
(d) Name two other causes of deformity of legs.

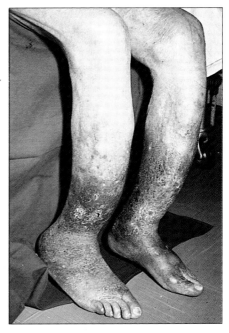

Question 127

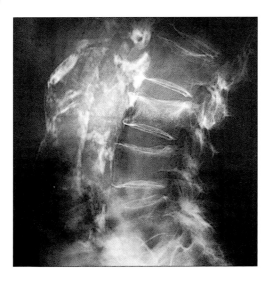

(a) What does the X-ray of abdomen show?
(b) What may be the clinical features?
(c) How would you confirm the diagnosis?
(d) What is the treatment?

Question 128

(a) What is the abnormality?
(b) Name three other sites where this kind of abnormality may be seen.

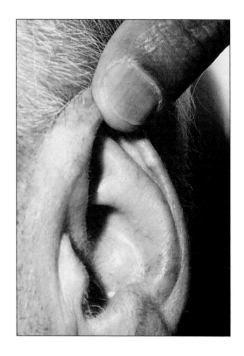

Question 129

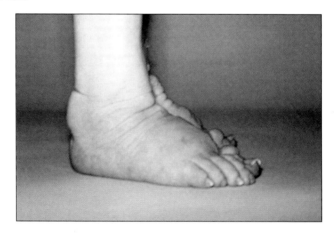

(a) What are the clinical features seen?
(b) What is the diagnosis?
(c) What is the underlying disease in which this abnormality may be found?

Question 130

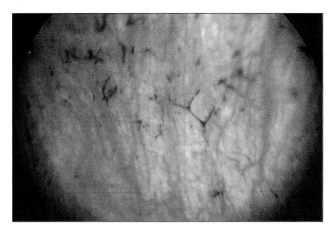

(a) What does this show?
(b) Name three features of this condition.
(c) What is the inheritance?

Question 131

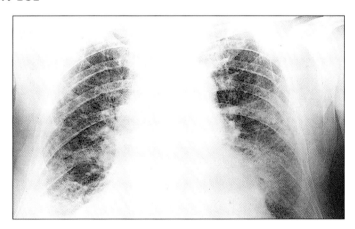

(a) What does this X-ray show?
(b) Name three features of this condition.
(c) Name three underlying causes giving rise to this condition.

Question 132

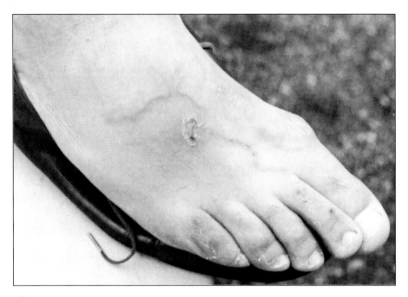

(a) What does this show?
(b) What are the best-known agents of this lesion?
(c) What may be the complication of this?

Question 133

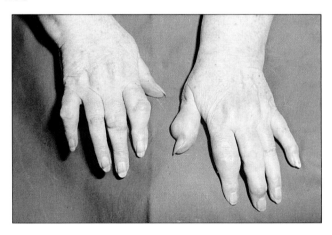

(a) What feature is this?
(b) How can the diagnosis be confirmed?
(c) Name four drugs commonly used for treatment of this condition.

Question 134

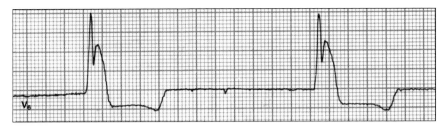

(a) What abnormalities are seen on this ECG?
(b) What may be the likely cause?

Question 135

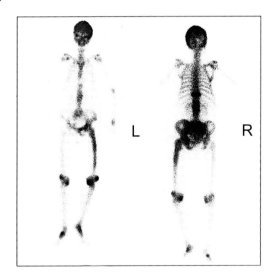

(a) What does this bone scan show?
(b) What is the likely diagnosis?

Question 136

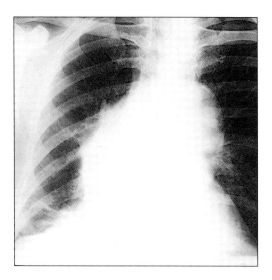

(a) What does this X-ray show?
(b) Name three likely causes.
(c) What further investigation should be carried out?

Question 137

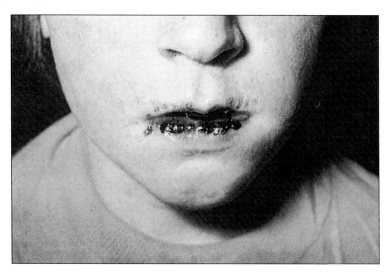

(a) What is this feature?
(b) Name two precipitating causes.
(c) Name four other sites of this lesion.

Question 138

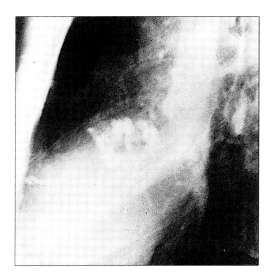

(a) What does this lateral view chest X-ray show?
(b) What does it indicate?
(c) What other non-invasive investigation would you like to carry out in this condition?

Question 139

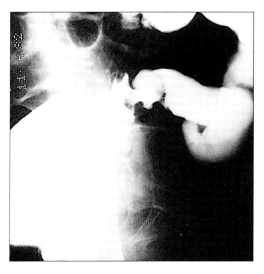

(a) What does this barium enema show?
(b) Name two clinical features of this condition.

Question 140

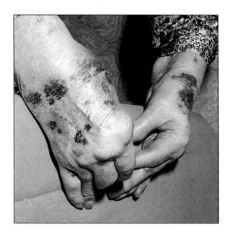

(a) What are the abnormalities shown?
(b) What may be the cause?

Question 141

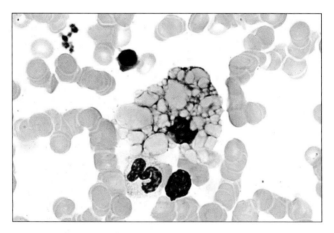

(a) What does this smear of bone marrow aspirate show?
(b) What disease does it indicate?
(c) What are the clinical types of this disease?

Question 142

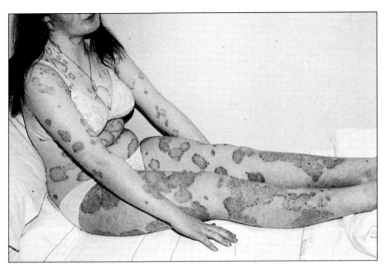

(a) What is this skin lesion shown in a girl of 16 years?
(b) What is the usual distribution of this skin lesion?
(c) Name two other features of this disease which may be found in much older patients.
(d) What is the treatment?

Question 143

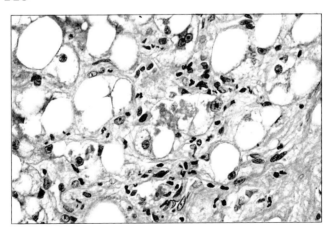

A 51-year-old female with a history of excessive alcohol intake presented with malnutrition, jaundice and hepatomegaly.
(a) What does this biopsy show?
(b) What is the diagnosis?

Question 144

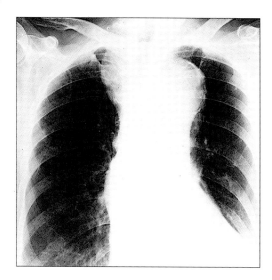

(a) Name two features shown on this chest X-ray.
(b) What is the most common cause?
(c) Name two features of this condition.

Question 145

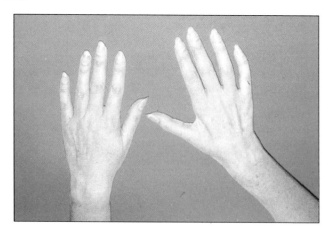

(a) What abnormality is seen in this patient?
(b) What is the likely diagnosis?
(c) Name two causes of this condition.

Question 146

(a) What is the abnormality?
(b) What is the likely diagnosis?
(c) Name three other features of this condition.
(d) What other investigation should be carried out?

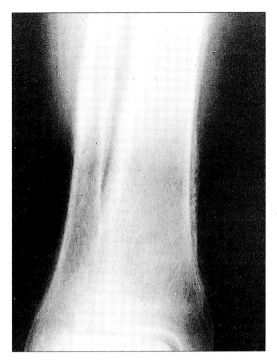

Question 147

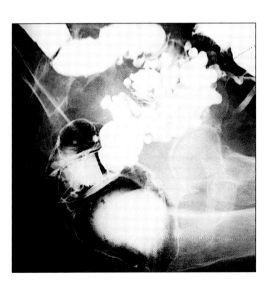

(a) What does this X-ray show?
(b) What are the common symptoms of uncomplicated lesion?
(c) What may be the complications of this condition?

Question 148

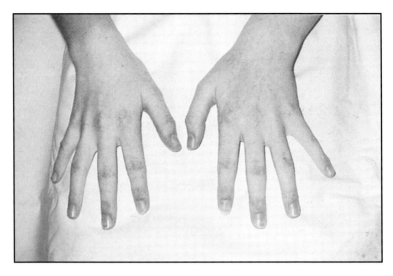

(a) What is the abnormality shown in this girl's hands?
(b) What may be the most common first symptom in this girl?
(c) What is the sex predilection in this disease and what is the mean age of onset of childhood?

Question 149

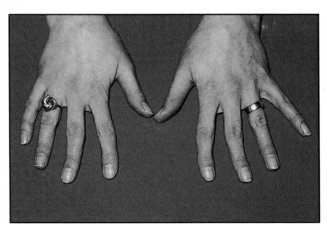

(a) What is the abnormality shown?
(b) What is the likely diagnosis?
(c) What is the inheritance?
(d) Name four other features of this condition.

Question 150

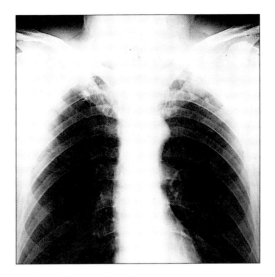

(a) What does this chest X-ray show?
(b) What is the diagnosis?

Question 151

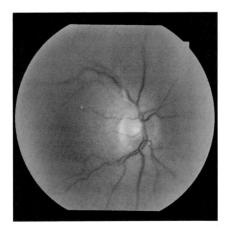

(a) What features are shown?
(b) What are the likely underlying causes?
(c) How does this affect the patient?

Question 152

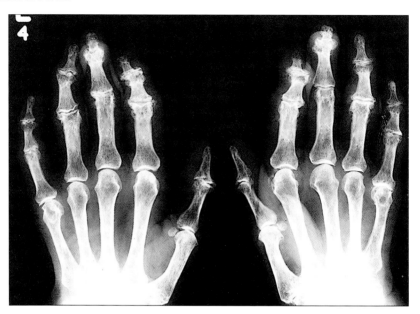

(a) What does this X-ray show?
(b) What is the likely diagnosis?

Question 153

(a) What are the ECG changes shown opposite and what are they likely to be due to?
(b) What conditions can give rise to this?
(c) Name three clinical features of this condition.

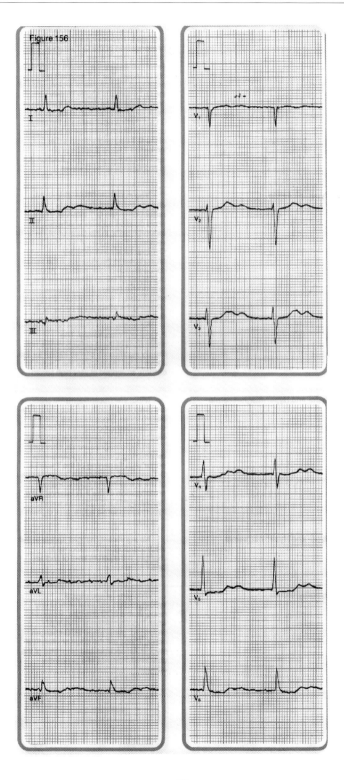

Figure 156

Question 154

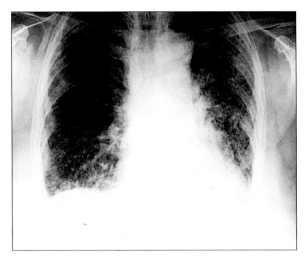

(a) What does this X-ray show?
(b) What is the likely diagnosis?
(c) Name three features of this condition.

Question 155

(a) What is this lesion on the leg of a
    32-year-old man?
(b) Which condition is this lesion
    associated with?

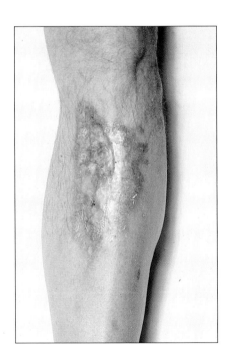

Question 156

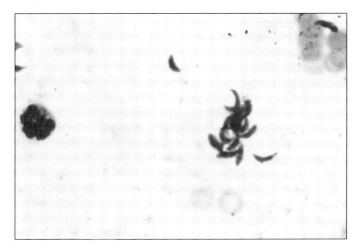

(a) What does this bone marrow show?
(b) How is the infection acquired?
(c) Name two eye conditions which may be caused by this infection.

Question 157

(a) What does this X-ray show?
(b) Name three features of this condition.
(c) Name four extra-articular manifestations of this condition.

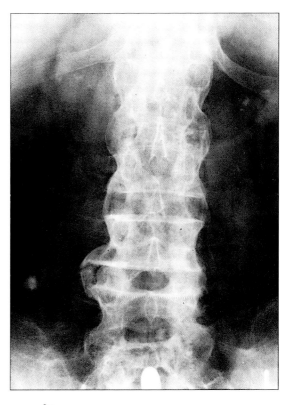

Question 158

(a) What abnormalities are seen
    in this girl of eleven years?
(b) Name two possible underlying
    conditions.

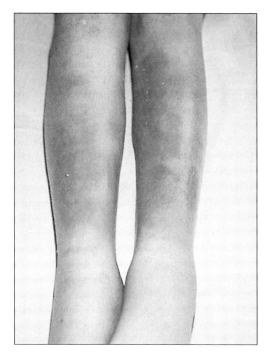

Question 159

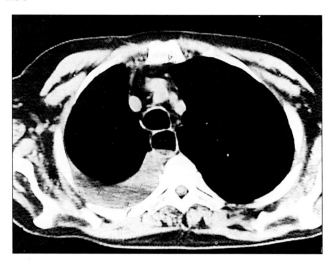

(a) What does this scan show?
(b) Name four common causes of this condition.

Question 160

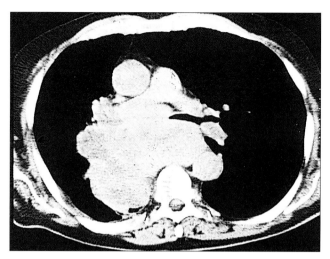

(a) What does this CT scan of the chest show?
(b) Name three causes for this.

Answers

Answer 1
(a) There is an extensive maculopapular rash on the lateral aspects of the back and on the right buttock.
(b) The likely cause is drug rash due to penicillin (ampicillin). A small percentage of patients may develop this kind of rash (approximately 5%).
(c) Hypersensitivity reactions are the most common adverse effects of penicillin which include fever, bronchospasm, vasculitis and anaphylaxis.

Answer 2
(a) Paget's disease of the skull.
(b) Serum alkaline phosphatase, urinary hydroxyproline and bone scan.

Answer 3
(a) This shows a Baker's cyst (in association with a large joint effusion).
(b) It may be confused with deep vein thrombosis of the leg.
(c) Ultrasonography may help in the diagnosis (see below).

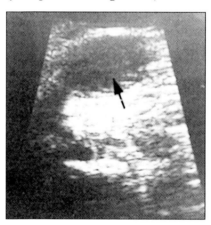

Answer 4
(a) The angiogram demonstrates a large right-sided posterior communicating artery aneurysm.
(b) Aneurysm of posterior communicating artery (if large) usually causes paralysis of the third cranial nerve and possibly hemianopia due to compression of the optic tract. There may also be sudden rupture leading to subarachnoid haemorrhage.
(c) CT scan is helpful but angiography is necessary for establishing the diagnosis and localization of the aneurysm prior to neurosurgery.

Answer 5

(a) Renal caseation and destruction of left kidney – parenchymal tissue is replaced by a mass of granulomatous tissue with extensive destruction of the normal renal parenchyma (autonephrectomy); also note large osteophytes in the vertebrae.

(b) Tuberculous infection of the kidney which occurred when the patient was much younger (now she is asymptomatic).

(c) The diagnosis of renal tuberculosis is made by:
  (i) Radiographic examination of the urinary tract
  (ii) Cystoscopy
  (iii) Demonstration of tubercle bacilli by cultures of the first morning voided urine.

Answer 6

(a) Right bundle branch block, left anterior hemiblock and 1st degree heart block (trifascicular block).

(b) Myocardial infarction.

(c) Implantation of pacemaker.

Answer 7

(a) The disc spaces of C5/6/7 are completely reduced with extensive degenerative osteophytes on the vertebral margins due to cervical spondylosis.

(b) Cervical radiculopathy, i.e. pain in the neck, pins and needles in the hands with impairment of reflexes in the upper limbs, and cervical myelopathy, i.e. weakness and spasticity of lower limbs with increased reflexes and extensor plantar response.

Answer 8

(a) Optic atrophy – note that the optic disc is pale and the margins are clear.

(b) Previous optic neuritis, previous disc oedema from raised intracranial pressure, chronic optic nerve compression and chronic glaucoma.

Answer 9

(a) A gastric ulcer in the lesser curvature.

(b) Pain in the epigastrium (not relieved by food), anorexia and loss of weight.

(c) Barium meal examination but endoscopy is preferred because it is more accurate and suspicious lesions can be biopsied for histological examination.

Answer 10

(a) The smear shows a typical 'hairy cell'.

(b) 'Hairy cell' leukaemia is commoner in males (M:F, 4:1). The patient complains of general debility, has recurrent infection, may have abdominal discomfort due to (gross) splenomegaly and hepatomegaly and there is usually pancytopenia due to hypersplenism and bone marrow infiltration or fibrosis.

Answer 11

(a) Sclerotic lesions are seen, more marked in the left ischium and to a lesser extent in the right superior pubic ramus – osteoblastic metastases from prostatic carcinoma.
(b) Symptoms of urethral obstruction, haematuria and bone pain.
(c) A clinical suspicion of prostatic cancer needs histological verification by needle biopsy. In addition, measurement of serum acid phosphatase and bone scan should be carried out.

Answer 12

(a) Hereditary haemorrhagic telangiectasia (Osler–Weber–Rendu disease). The diagnosis is made in the setting of repeated episodes of bleeding, the presence of multiple telangiectases, and a positive family history.
(b) It is transmitted as an autosomal dominant trait.
(c) Mucous membrane bleeding, particularly epistaxis, is the commonest presentation.

Answer 13

(a) Vasospastic changes induced by cold water immersion.
(b) This feature is seen in systemic lupus erythematosus.

Answer 14

(a) Trypanomastigote of *Trypanosoma cruzi*.
(b) American trypanosomiasis (Chagas' disease).
(c) Transmitted to man from the faeces of a reduviid bug in which the trypanosomes have a cycle of development before becoming infective to man.

Answer 15

(a) Calcification of the pericardium due to constrictive pericarditis.
(b) A raised jugulo-venous pressure, pulsus paradoxus, and hepatomegaly with ascites (without enlargement of heart and peripheral oedema).
(c) Surgical resection of the pericardium.

Answer 16

(a) A generalized metallic grey-brown hyperpigmentation of skin is seen in this patient (only the face and lower limbs are shown here).

(b) Idiopathic haemochromatosis.

(c) Autosomal recessive inheritance.

(d) Liver biopsy to confirm iron overload to assess tissue damage.

Answer 17

(a) 'Pencil-in-cup' deformity of the proximal interphalangeal joint.

(b) Psoriatic arthropathy.

Answer 18

(a) This CT scan shows an abnormal round dense lesion in the left mid-parietal area.

(b) Meningioma.

(c) CT scan is usually diagnostic and angiography often demonstrates filling of the tumour from the meningeal circulation and vascular displacement.

Answer 19

(a) (i) Koilonychia – flattening or concavity of three nails.
    (ii) Heberden's nodes.

(b) Iron deficiency anaemia.

(c) Microcytosis, hypochromasia, poikilocytosis and a low mean cell volume (MCV).

Answer 20

(a) There is a considerable bulge to the mid-left ventricular border.

(b) Left ventricular aneurysm.

(c) Acute myocardial infarction.

(d) A sizeable ventricular aneurysm may result in congestive cardiac failure, ventricular arrhythmias or mural thrombosis (and systemic embolization).

Answer 21

(a) Complete right third cranial nerve palsy.

(b) Look for evidence of complete internal ophthalmoplegia (i.e. widely dilated pupil which fails to react to light and accomodation and the patient is unable to move the eye in any direction except outwards).

(c) A unilateral third-nerve palsy developing rapidly with pain behind the eye commonly occurs due to a supraclinoid aneurysm of the internal carotid artery or posterior communicating artery; the other two possible causes of complete nerve palsy are a tumour and diabetes mellitus.

(d) CT scan and carotid angiography (if neurosurgery is contemplated).

Answer 22

(a) Slide of a bone marrow showing abnormal plasma cells with eccentric nucleus, prominent nucleoli and deep blue cytoplasm.

(b) Multiple myeloma.

(c) Bone pain, anaemia, recurrent infection and pathological fractures.

(d) Plasma viscoity (very high), serum electrophoresis, immunoglobulins and complete skeletal radiological survey.

Answer 23

(a) Asymmetrical polyarthritis mainly involving the distal interphalangeal joints of both hands and metacarpophalangeal joint of right index finger (and to a lesser extent of the left index finger), erythematous scaly skin lesions over the extensor surface of both hands and nail changes including pitting and onycholysis.

(b) Psoriatic arthropathy.

(c) Negative tests for rheumatoid factor (and antinuclear factor), and radiographs showing asymmetrical disease with terminal interphalangeal joint involvement and almost no periarticular osteoporosis.

Answer 24

(a) The scan shows that the anterior part of the left renal cortex is expanded with a slightly irregular outline which is very likely due to carcinoma (the other possibility is xanthogranulomatous pyelonephritis)

(b) Renal colic and a palpable mass in the flank.

(c) IVU with nephrotomography, chest X-ray (to exclude metastasis in the chest) and radionuclide bone scan.

Answer 25

(a) Prognathos (due to overgrowth of the mandible), coarsened features resulting from soft tissue hypertrophy with thickening of skin folds of the face and enlargement of lower lip.

(b) Acromegaly.

(c) Large hands (necessitating ring enlargement and increased glove size), enlarged tongue and hypertension (with cardiomegaly).

(d) The diagnosis is confirmed by measuring growth hormone levels (high) during an oral glucose tolerance test.

Answer 26

(a) Right bundle branch block and atrial flutter.

(b) (i) Right bundle branch block – congenital heart disease (ASD) and coronary artery disease.

(ii) Atrial flutter – coronary artery disease (acute myocardial infarction) and rheumatic mitral valve disease.

Answer 27

(a) This liver biopsy shows chronic inflammatory cells, mainly lymphocytes and plasma cells, aggressively destroying the limiting plate (which runs horizontally across the field) and apparently attacking periportal hepatocytes which show ballooning degeneration.

(b) Chronic active hepatitis, piecemeal necrosis.

Answer 28

(a) Lymphoedema due to Milroy's disease.

(b) Lymphoedema due to filariasis and obstruction of the lymphatics by tumour cells.

Answer 29

(a) Wasting of small muscles of both hands, loss of distal part of right thumb and right index fingers and trophic lesions in the right index and middle fingers.

(b) Syringomyelia.

(c) Dissociated sensory loss (i.e. loss of pain and temperature sensation but appreciation of light touch and postural sensibility are preserved), loss of reflexes in the upper limb and upper motor signs in the legs, dysarthria, nystagmus and Horner's syndrome.

(d) Motor neurone disease, cervical spondylosis and tumour of the spinal cord.

Answer 30

(a) Megaloblasts in the smear of bone marrow aspirate of a patient suffering from vitamin B12-deficiency anaemia.

(b) Intrinsic factor antibody and Schilling test.

Answer 31

(a) Blue-grey sclerae.

(b) Osteogenesis imperfecta.

(c) Multiple pathological fractures.

Answer 32

(a) X-ray (i) shows patchy consolidation of right base and pleurally based soft tissue mass in the mid-axillary line (R) and X-ray (ii) shows destruction of (absent) pedicle of L2.

(b) Right basal pneumonia and multiple metastases from possibly bronchogenic carcinoma.

Answer 33

(a) Microfilaria of *Wuchereria bancrofti* in blood smear. The sheath is clearly visible. The dark dots are nuclei.

(b) *Wuchereria bancrofti* is commonly conveyed to man by the bites of the infected mosquito – *Culex fatigans*.

(c) Bouts of fever accompanied by pain, tenderness and erythema along the course of inflamed lymphatic vessels, regional lymph node enlargement and elephantiasis.

Answer 34

(a) Horner's syndrome.

(b) Ptosis (partial), miosis and ipsilateral anhydrosis (due to interruption of sympathetic pathways).

(c) Internal carotid artery occlusion, bronchogenic carcinoma (Pancoast tumour) and syringomyelia.

Answer 35

(a) Pigmentation of the lips and extensive abnormal calcification of the right suprarenal gland.

(b) Addison's disease.

(c) Tuberculosis, metastatic carcinoma and autoimmune adrenalitis.

(d) Weight loss, vomiting and hypotension.

Answer 36

(a) (i) Wolff–Parkinson–White syndrome. This ECG was taken during sinus rhythm. This syndrome is characterized by a short P–R interval, a widened QRS complex due to the presence of delta wave (and a tendency to paroxysmal tachycardia).

    (ii) Wolff–Parkinson–White syndrome. This ECG was taken during atrial fibrillation. The ventricular rate is rapid and irregular. The QRS complexes are abnormally wide. This is atrial fibrillation with atrioventricular conduction occurring via the anomalous atrioventricular pathway.

(b) This syndrome is caused by an accessory connection between atrial and ventricular myocardium.

(c) Very rapid ventricular rate (sometimes ventricular fibrillation and death) and atrial fibrillation which is a particularly dangerous event.

(d) Disopyramide quinidine or amiodarone.

Answer 37

(a) The first metatarsophalangeal joint of the big toe is red and swollen with shiny overlying skin; similar changes are also seen in the adjoining tissues of the foot.

(b) Acute gout.

(c) The onset may be explosively sudden, often waking the patient from sleep.

(d) Colchicine, indomethacin and ibuprofen.

Answer 38

(a) Multiple small tumours visible in the skin and café-au-lait patches.

(b) Neurofibromatosis.

(c) It is inherited as an autosomal dominant.

(d) Phaeochromocytoma, congenital bone abnormalities, and tumours of brain (spinal cord and peripheral nerves).

Answer 39

(a) Exophthalmos (bilateral).

(b) Thyrotoxicosis, retro-orbital tumours and Paget's disease of bone.

Answer 40

(a) X-ray (i) shows distortion of the duodenal cap, and X-ray (ii) shows duodenal ulcer.

(b) Barium meal examination; if a duodenal ulcer is demonstrated radiologically, no further diagnostic test is necessary. However, if symptoms fail to subside following adequate therapy, endoscopy may be required.

(c) Famotidine and omeprazole.

Answer 41

(a) Cutaneous anthrax on the neck. The lesion begins as an itching papule which enlarges and forms a vesicle filled with serosanguineous fluid surrounded by marked oedema. The vesicle dries up to form a thick black 'eschar' surrounded by blebs. There may be some enlargement of the regional lymph nodes.

(b) Humans may contract the disease by close contact with infected domestic animals, or by eating the flesh of animals that have died from anthrax.

(c) (i) When the sore is on the neck, the oedema may encircle the neck and press on the trachea or sometimes there is oedema of the larynx giving rise to difficulty in breathing, needing tracheostomy as a life-saving measure.

(ii) Meningitis.

(d) Benzylpenicillin, 2400–3600 mg/day iv for about 12 days.

Answer 42

(a) This shows diabetic retinopathy with hard exudates, haemorrhages and microaneurysms.

(b) Soft exudates, neovascularization, vitreous haemorrhage and fibrovascular membrane.

Answer 43

(a) Clubbing of fingers and toes.
(b) Clubbing results from oedema, cellular infiltration, and connective tissue proliferation in the nail beds.
(c) Bronchogenic carcinoma, cyanotic heart disease, bronchiectasis and bacterial endocarditis.

Answer 44

(a) The ECG recording is from a patient with mirror-image dextrocardia ('situs inversion'), lead I shows an inverted P wave, QRS complex and T wave which is a very unusual finding. The appearances in V1 are consistent with normality but from V2–V6 the r waves become progressively smaller than larger and there is T wave inversion.
(b) There is no evidence of organic heart disease.
(c) The patient was probably born with left–right inversion of the body organs.

Answer 45

(a) (i) Discoid and (ii) butterfly lesions of systemic lupus erythematosus.
(b) Arthritis, arthralgia and fever.
(c) The presence of large amounts of antibodies to native DNA is the single most useful diagnostic laboratory finding.

Answer 46

(a) Gynaecomastia (usually results from an increased circulating oestrogen level relative to the testosterone level).
(b) Bronchogenic carcinoma, hepatic cirrhosis, prostatic carcinoma, drugs (e.g. digoxin and spironolactone) and Klinefelter's syndrome.

Answer 47

(a) Severe kyphosis – gibbous deformity (hunchback deformity).
(b) Tuberculosis of the thoracic spine (Pott's disease). Characteristically, the infection starts at the margins of the vertebral bodies with subsequent invasion of the disc space. Destruction of bone leads to angular kyphosis.
(c) Tuberculosis became rare in the West but there is evidence of a recent increase in the elderly population.

Answer 48

(a) Multiple rounded shadows due to secondaries in the lungs.
(b) Bronchogenic, breast and bowel carcinoma.

Answer 49

(a) The X-ray shows numerous cysticercus cellulosae in the skeletal musculature of both forearms.

(b) When superficially placed, cysts can be felt under the skin or mucosa as pea-like ovoid bodies, epilepsy, staggering gait and hydrocephalus.

(c) Calcified cysts in the muscles can be seen radiologically (as seen in this X-ray) but they may not be visible when situated in the central nervous system; computed tomography should demonstrate these lesions.

Answer 50

(a) (i) This shows poorly defined areas of non-enhancement of the anterior portion of the body of the pancreas due to neoplasm.

(ii) It also shows an area of non-enhancement of water density in the left kidney due to a simple cyst.

(b) Abdominal pain, loss of weight and progressive (painless) jaundice.

(c) Liver function tests, glucose tolerance tests, barium meal (or endoscopy) and ultrasonography.

Answer 51

(a) Erythema ab igne.

(b) It occurs due to the patient sitting too near the fire and for too long. This results in intense vasodilation, red cell leakage from capillaries and skin staining with iron deposits.

(c) Elderly people are prone to develop this because of reduced sensory feeling, and increased need for external warmth (using electric bar fires and open coal fires).

Answer 52

(a) The carotid angiogram shows a tight stenosis at the origin of the internal carotid artery.

(b) Monoocular visual symptoms, paresis (mono-, hemi-), paraesthesia (mono-, hemi-) and facial paresis.

(c) Carotid endarterectomy reduces the risk of stroke and death in patients with severe stenosis (greater than 70%) of the cervical portion of the internal carotid artery who are experiencing transient hemispheric or retinal ischaemia and these patients are likely to benefit from surgery.

Answer 53

(a) Swan neck deformity with hyperextension of the proximal interphalangeal joint and flexion of the distal interphalangeal joint due to rheumatoid arthritis.

(b) Joint pain, stiffness and symmetrical swelling of a number of peripheral joints.

(c) Subcutaneous nodules, Sjögren's syndrome, popliteal cysts (Baker's cysts), and vasculitis.

Answer 54

(a) Hypertensive retinopathy, showing A/V nipping and tortuosity of vessels temporal to the disc, may be seen after venous occlusion.
(b) With more severe hypertension, retinal haemorrhages, exudates and papilloedema may occur. In early retinopathy, there is little or no effect on visual acuity. However, extensive haemorrhages or exudates can cause visual field defects or blindness if the macula is affected.

Answer 55

(a) This shows multiple giant cell granuloma in bone biopsy of a patient with sarcoidosis.
(b) Chest radiograph may show bilateral symmetrical hilar adenopathy often associated with paratracheal adenopathy. Computed tomographic (CT) scan can demonstrate lymphadenopathy more clearly and, in particular, can detect anterior mediastinal and subcarinal lymph nodes that have gone undetected on conventional films of the chest.

Answer 56

(a) Z deformity of the thumbs and gross deformity of hands with ulnar deviation.
(b) Rheumatoid arthritis.

Answer 57

(a) Mitral annular calcification; it has a C-shaped configuration and lies in the region of the mitral valve.
(b) Mitral valve calcification; an easy distinction is based on its configuration.
(c) It may be associated with dysrhythmias and systemic emboli.

Answer 58

(a) Grossly enlarged lateral ventricles, cortical atrophy and widened sulci.
(b) Dementia due to Alzheimer's disease.
(c) Loss of general intelligence, memory impairment, personality change and emotional changes (in advanced dementia, emotional reaction becomes blunted).
(d) Chest X-ray, serum B12 and thyroid function tests.

Answer 59

(a) Bony swellings in the distal interphalangeal joints with flexor and lateral deviations of the distal phalanx of the index and middle fingers.
(b) Heberden's nodes (osteoarthritis).

(c) Pain in the affected joints, increased by activity of the joints and morning stiffness.

Answer 60

(a) Punched out lesions in the skull.

(b) Multiple myeloma.

(c) Anaemia, renal failure, recurrent infection and amyloidosis.

Answer 61

(a) Atrial flutter with complete heart block. On this ECG complete heart block can only be diagnosed by the finding of a regular, very slow (usually 50 beats/min or less) ventricular rate in the presence of atrial flutter.

(b) Atrial flutter with complete heart block is not a common combination, in most cases of atrial flutter there is 2:1, 3:1, 4:1 or 5:1 atrioventricular block with corresponding ventricular rate of 150, 100, 75 or 60 beats/min.

Answer 62

(a) This shows characteristic pigmented spots over lips due to Peutz–Jeghers syndrome.

(b) Polyposis of the small (and/or large) bowel is part of the syndrome.

Answer 63

(a) A large head due to Paget's disease of skull.

(b) Bone pain, deafness and deformity of legs.

(c) Calcitonin, diphosphonates and mithramycin.

Answer 64

(a) Staghorn calculus (in the right kidney) due to hyperparathyroidism.

(b) Raised serum calcium and raised PTH.

(c) Demineralization and subperiosteal erosions in the phalanges, a 'pepper-pot' appearance seen on lateral radiographs of the skull and nephrocalcinosis (scattered opacities within the renal outline).

Answer 65

(a) This is a smear of aspirate of a patient with sideroblastic myelodysplastic syndrome, illustrating ringed sideroblasts.

(b) Sideroblastic anaemia is usually divided into two groups: (i) acquired – the anaemia develops insidiously and is often discovered during a routine examination; (ii) hereditary sideroblastic anaemia is almost always a disease of males and is probably inherited as an X-linked recessive trait.

Answer 66

(a) Bilateral hilar lymphadenopathy.

(b) Sarcoidosis and Hodgkin's disease.

Answer 67

(a) A large area of macular degeneration; there is also an area of atrophy around the optic disc.

(b) Visual field defects or blindness.

Answer 68

(a) This shows acne vulgaris.

(b) This is common between the ages of fourteen and nineteen years.

(c) (i) Topical treatment – benzoyl peroxide and retinoic acid creams.
    (ii) Oral tetracyclines.

Answer 69

(a) This shows abnormal patchy shadowing (large dense masses) present in each upper and mid zone with emphysema in each lower zone due to pneumoconiosis with progressive massive fibrosis.

(b) Pulmonary tuberculosis.

Answer 70

(a) Generalized osteoporosis with collapse of many vertebrae.

(b) Low backache (most common), kyphosis (with loss of height), fracture of the vertebrae, hips and wrists.

(c) Single and dual photon absorptiometry, quantitative computed tomography using single energy scanning and iliac trephine biopsy (to exclude osteomalacia in doubtful cases).

Answer 71

(a) Flexion contracture, loss of skin creases and tight waxy appearance of skin of hands.

(b) Sclerodactyly.

(c) Hypomotility of the oesophagus (demonstrated by barium swallow examination) and pulmonary fibrosis.

Answer 72

(a) Collapse of D12 (vertebra).

(b) Osteoporosis, multiple myeloma and metastatic deposit.

(c) Backache.

(d) (i) Serum calcium and alkaline phosphatase.
    (ii) Plasma viscosity.

(iii) Plasma protein (electrophoresis).

(iv) Sternal marrow examination.

(v) Chest X-ray.

Answer 73

(a) Left facial palsy – lower motor neurone lesion.

(b) Bell's palsy.

(c) Within the facial canal.

(d) Multiple sclerosis and 'geniculate' herpes zoster (Ramsay–Hunt syndrome).

Answer 74

(a) Liver biopsy shows that the epithelium of the interlobular bile duct on the left of the field has been almost totally destroyed; it is surrounded by inflammatory cells which are predominantly lymphocytes and plasma cells. To the right of the duct is a large ill-defined epitheloid granuloma.

(b) Primary biliary cirrhosis.

(c) Weight loss, hepatomegaly and splenomegaly.

Answer 75

(a) Rheumatoid nodules.

(b) They are almost invariably associated with seropositive (rheumatoid factor) disease and perhaps with a more severe and destructive arthritis.

(c) The olecranon bursae, extensor surface of the forearms, and the achilles tendon.

(d) Histological appearance is that of a central necrotic area surrounded by palisades of fibroblasts, histiocytes and macrophages.

Answer 76

(a) Absence of axillary hair and enlarged pituitary fossa.

(b) Hypopituitarism (pituitary tumour).

(c) Characteristically finer and more wrinkled skin (premature aging), gynaecomastia and small softened testicles.

Answer 77

(a) This cervical myelogram shows obstruction, at the level of C3/C4.

(b) Cervical myelopathy due to cervical spondylosis and obstruction due to tumour.

(c) Magnetic resonance imaging.

Answer 78

(a) Two small lumps in the skin of the back due to secondaries.

(b) Carcinoma of lung, breast or bowel.

(c) Examination for a breast lump (and biopsy of the lump), X-ray of the chest, barium enema; but biopsy of the skin lump will be the simplest way of establishing the diagnosis.

Answer 79

(a) Large ulcerative lesions of the nose due to mucocutaneous leishmaniasis.

(b) *Leishmania braziliensis.*

(c) Reservoir hosts for *L. braziliensis* are rodents, certain wild animal species and more rarely dogs. Vectors are females of sandfly species belonging to the genus *Phebotomus.*

Answer 80

(a) Atrial flutter with varying AV block. The QRS rate is irregular and there is no clearly recognizable pattern in the P–R interval. The QRS complexes are narrow and the rhythm is clearly supraventricular. Flutter waves are clearly recognizable. The degree of AV block varies.

(b) With a regular 2:1 AV block, it may be difficult to distinguish atrial flutter from supraventricular or sinus tachycardia; carotid sinus pressure may help by temporarily increasing the degree of block.

Answer 81

(a) Type 1 second degree atrioventricular block (Wenckebach second degree block, Mobitz type 1 second degree block). The condition is usually recognized in the context of normal background sinus activation of the atria and there is a progressive prolongation of the P–R interval (with each successive beat) until one P wave fails to be followed by a QRS complex. Following this dropped beat the P–R interval usually shortens abruptly and the cycle starts all over again.

(b) This is due to progressive fatigue of the AV bundle with recovery following the rest period when the dropped beat occurs.

Answer 82

(a) Microstomia, perioral skin puckering and telangiectasia.

(b) Systemic sclerosis.

(c) Raynaud's phenomenon.

Answer 83

(a) This shows circular, well-defined areas of iso-echogenic areas with a hypo-echogenic border (target lesions) – a typical picture of (multiple) secondary deposits.

(b) Bronchogenic carcinoma, carcinoma of the bowel and breast.

Answer 84
(a) Palmar erythema and ulnar deviation of the fingers.
(b) Rheumatoid arthritis.

Answer 85
(a) Swelling of the ankle joint due to neuropathic joint disease (Charcot joint).
(b) Diabetes mellitus.
(c) Syringomyelia and syphilitic tabes dorsalis.

Answer 86
(a) Hiatus hernia.
(b) (i) Heart burn – occurs usually after meals and characteristically is brought on by bending down or straining, due to an increased intra-abdominal pressure, or lying down.
   (ii) Dysphagia.
   (iii) Anaemia.
(c) Barium swallow, but endoscopy is the preferred investigation.

Answer 87
(a) This shows Henoch–Schonlein purpura (purpura over buttocks is florid).
(b) This is an allergic vasculitis and the most common childhood vasculitis.
(c) Abdominal colic, intussusception, vomiting and transient haematuria.

Answer 88
(a) Increased markings, patchy infiltrates and ring shadows in both lung bases.
(b) Bronchiectasis.
(c) Copious sputum, haemoptysis and finger clubbing.
(d) Bronchography is the definitive procedure to establish the diagnosis and determine the extent and distribution of lesions. It is indicated only in patients who are likely to undergo surgery.

Answer 89
(a) Bony enlargement with deformity affecting the proximal interphalangeal joints of almost all the fingers – due to Bouchard's nodes (in addition, note Heberden's nodes in all the fingers).
(b) Osteoarthritis.

Answer 90
(a) Herpes zoster – note dermatomal distribution.

(b) This condition is the result of reactivation of varicella zoster virus, which has lain dormant in a posterior nerve root ganglion following infection with the chickenpox virus earlier in life.

(c) Post-hepatic neuralgia, segmental muscle wasting from involvement of the motor root (uncommon) and encephalitis (occasionally).

(d) Idoxuridine may be applied to the skin in a 5% solution initially. Oral acyclovir 200 mg, 5 times a day for 5 to 10 days, is useful if started early.

Answer 91

(a) Retinal scars following treatment of diabetic retinopathy (pan photocoagulation) with laser.

(b) Diabetic retinopathy is the most common cause of blindness between the ages of 30 and 65, in the Western world. Retinal photocoagulation is an effective treatment if it is given early when the patient is usually asymptomatic (regular ophthalmoscopy for all diabetic patients is mandatory).

Answer 92

(a) Extensive nodular shadowing most marked in the upper and mid zones.

(b) Old miliary tuberculosis and coal miner's pneumoconiosis (grade 3).

Answer 93

(a) Right ventricular hypertrophy with acute pericarditis. The record shows sinus rhythm. There is widespread ST segment elevation indicative of acute pericarditis. The form of the QRS complexes in V1 is indicative of right ventrical hypertrophy.

(b) The patient has an atrial septal defect and developed pericarditis as an immediate reaction to the operation.

Answer 94

(a) Large, fleshy hands (spade-like).

(b) Acromegaly.

(c) Other causes of enlargement of hands are hypothyroidism, manual work, primary amyloidosis and obesity.

Answer 95

(a) Note contracture of medial three fingers, due to Dupuytren's contracture.

(b) The earliest abnormality in Dupuytren's contracture is the formation of fibrous nodules, probably resulting from contraction of proliferative fibroblasts in the superficial compartment of the palm. Later, contracture is caused by a thickening and shortening of the palmar facia.

(c) The exact causes are not known but occupation, heredity and cirrhosis of liver are thought to be possible predisposing factors.

(d) The disorder is about five times more prevalent in males than in females.

Answer 96

(a) Deformity of left thigh and lengthening of right leg.

(b) Paget's disease of bone.

(c) X-ray of left thigh and right leg (see X-ray below) and estimation of serum alkaline phosphatase.

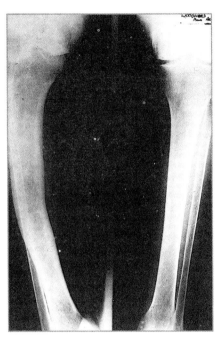

Answer 97

(a) This shows an opacity (and cardiomegaly) at the right cardio-phrenic angle due to a pericardial cyst.

(b) A lateral chest X-ray should localize the lesion and no further investigations are usually required because this has no clinical significance.

(c) Hiatus hernia, paravertebral abscess, neurofibroma and bronchogenic carcinoma.

Answer 98

(a) Marked wasting of proximal muscles (particularly supraspinati, infraspinati and glutei).

(b) Thyrotoxicosis.

(c) Tachycardia, exophthalmos and heat intolerance.

(d) Estimation of serum T3, T4 and TSH.

Answer 99

(a) Tufting of terminal phalanges which is characteristic of acromegaly.

(b) In acromegaly, cartilage hypertrophy may also occur giving rise to widened joint spaces, most marked in the metacarpophalangeal joints (see X-ray below).

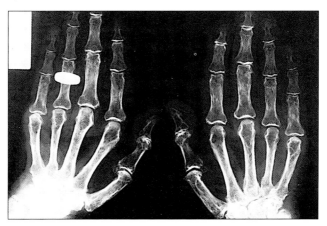

Answer 100

(a) This shows digital gangrene of the fingers of the left hand.

(b) Rheumatoid vasculitis – also note the deformity of the hands, particularly the right hand (due to rheumatoid arthritis).

Answer 101

(a) Xanthelasma.

(b) Hyperlipidaemia (hypercholesterolaemia).

(c) Ischaemic heart disease, but this is not necessarily indicative of severe hyperlipidaemia in the elderly.

Answer 102

(a) Wasting of small muscles of hand.

(b) Motor neurone disease.

Answer 103

(a) This CT scan of the brain shows a 5 cm ringed enhancing mass in the right fronto-parietal region surrounded by a great deal of oedema, causing contralateral shift of the lateral ventricles due to a metastatic lesion.

(b) X-ray of chest (see overleaf); shows a 5-cm diameter lobulated mass lesion due to a carcinoma in the right upper lobe.

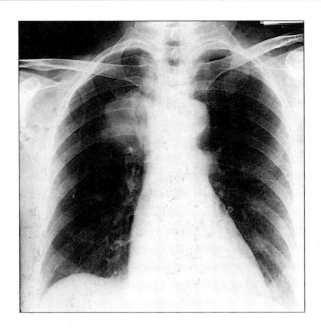

Answer 104

(a) Paget's disease of pelvis and right femur (with complete fracture), osteoarthritis of hip joints and triradiate deformity of pelvis.

(b) High-output cardiac failure, pathological fractures and osteogenic sarcoma.

(c) About 4% of people over 55 years old and of west European extraction (United Kingdom, United States, Canada, Australia and New Zealand) suffer from Paget's disease of bone.

Answer 105

(a) Exposure of the metatarsal heads due to metatarsophalangeal subluxation resulting in callus formation.

(b) Rheumatoid arthritis.

Answer 106

(a) The ultrasound scan shows the maximum transverse diameter of the abdominal aorta to be 3.8 cm (normal is up to 2.5 cm) – a small aneurysm of the abdominal aorta.

(b) The frequency of aneurysm of the abdominal aorta in men outnumbers that in women by 6:1.

(c) The risk of rupture is higher if the patient complains of pain in the lower back (a sign of enlargement of the aneurysm) or if the ultrasound demonstrates a lesion of 7 cm or larger.

Answer 107

(a) Marked cachexia (and nicotine stain of the finger) with clubbing.

(b) Bronchogenic carcinoma.

(c) Radiological examination of the chest (see below), examination of sputum for malignant cells and bronchoscopy (with biopsy).

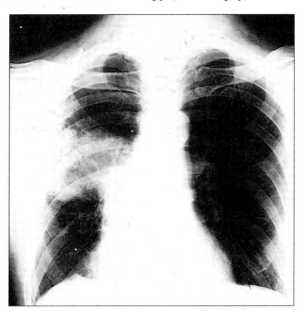

Answer 108

(a) Superior temporal vein branch occlusion showing haemorrhages and soft exudates.

(b) This condition should be distinguished from vasculitis.

(c) The patient complains of blurred vision.

Answer 109

(a) Destruction of the head of the first metatarsal and base of the adjacent phalanx (incidental amputation of the middle toe).

(b) Gout

Answer 110

(a) Thickening and tortuosity of the artery in the temple.

(b) Temporal (giant cell) arteritis.

(c) Headache, malaise and weight loss.

(d) Plasma viscosity (high) and temporal artery biopsy, which may show inflammatory infiltrate composed of histiocytes, lymphocytes and giant cells surrounding markedly fragmented internal elastic lamina, with intervening normal arterial segments.

Answer 111

(a) The radiograph shows calcium pyrophosphate dihydrate (CPPD) deposition in the menisci and articular cartilage in both knees – chondrocalcinosis.
(b) By examination of the synovial fluid under polarizing light microscopy which will show intraleukocytic positively birefringent crystals of CPPD.

Answer 112

(a) Bullous impetigo.
(b) Staphylococci and streptococci.

Answer 113

(a) Schizont of *Plasmodium vivax* (malaria parasite).
(b) Fever, enlargement of spleen (and liver) and anaemia.

Answer 114

(a) It shows 'hair on end' appearance of the skull.
(b) Thalassaemia major.
(c) Anaemia, retardation of development and growth, and splenomegaly.

Answer 115

(a) Marked pallor and a smooth tongue (glossitis).
(b) Addisonian pernicious anaemia.
(c) Macrocytic dysplastic blood picture, megablastic marrow, very low serum vitamin B12 (less than 50 ng/L), intrinsic factor antibodies in the serum and Schilling test.

Answer 116

(a) A secondary deposit, on the medial aspect of the left femur.
(b) Bronchogenic, breast or bowel carcinoma.

Answer 117

(a) Subdural haematoma (bilateral).
(b) Alcoholics, the elderly and patients receiving anticoagulants.
(c) Headache, fluctuating level of consciousness, confusion, memory loss and focal neurological deficit.

Answer 118
(a) Acute chondrocalcinosis – note swelling of the right hand.
(b) X-ray of the hand may show intra-articular calcification of the wrist joint.

Answer 119
(a) Marked yellow discolouration of the conjunctiva.
(b) Obstructive jaundice due to biliary stones, pancreatic carcinoma and metastatic tumours (intrahepatic).
(c) Liver function tests and abdominal ultrasound examination.

Answer 120
(a) Deformity of tibia and fibula of both legs of an adult (this deformity occurred when he was a child).
(b) Rickets (childhood) – due to vitamin D deficiency.
(c) (i) Bone pain.
   (ii) Reduction in growth and bowing of the long bones.
   (iii) Bossing of the frontal and parietal bones of the skull.
   (iv) Swelling of the costochondral junctions (rickety rosary).
(d) (i) Biochemical investigations (plasma calcium, plasma phosphate, alkaline phosphatase and $1,25(OH)_2D_3$.
   (ii) Radiological examination will show widening of the growth plate with a cupped and ragged metaphysis.

Answer 121
(a) Parkinson's disease.
(b) Tremor, rigidity and bradykinesia.
(c) Levodopa, levodopa plus carbidopa and selegiline.

Answer 122
(a) The X-ray shows right-sided pleural effusion.
(b) Ultrasonography, pleural aspiration (and biopsy), sputum (for tubercle bacilli and malignant cells) and bronchoscopy (with biopsy).

Answer 123
(a) Red to purple ecchymoses on the extensor surface of forearms and hands.
(b) Senile purpura.
(c) It results from degeneration and loss of collagen, elastin and subcutaneous fat in the skin; it usually occurs spontaneously but may also be precipitated by minor trauma.

Answer 124
(a) Left-sided pneumothorax (spontaneous).

(b) Rupture of a subpleural emphysematous bulla and rupture of a subpleural tuberculous focus into the pleural space.

(c) Cyanosis, hyper-resonant percussion note and diminished (or absent) breath sounds on the affected side.

Answer 125

(a) Bilateral wasting of muscles of the thenar eminence.

(b) Carpal tunnel syndrome.

(c) Paraesthesia in the radial three and a half digits of the hand, particularly at night, and nerve compression locally (Tinel's sign) can induce characteristic symptoms.

(d) Rheumatoid (or osteo) arthritis, pregnancy, hypothyroidism and amyloidosis.

Answer 126

(a) Anterior bowing of legs.

(b) Paget's disease.

(c) Usually there is no hypercalcaemia in this condition, but immobilization, e.g. following fracture of the neck of femur, can cause hypercalcaemia.

(d) Rickets in childhood and yaws.

Answer 127

(a) Calcification of aneurysm of abdominal aorta, partial collapse of L3 and generalized osteoporosis.

(b) Backache, intermittent claudication, or may be acute presentation with abdominal pain and hypotension as a result of rupture. Abdominal palpation will demonstrate an 'expansile' pulsation of the aneurysm.

(c) Abdominal ultrasound scanning followed by angiography.

(d) Elective surgical repair results in a much lower mortality than emergency surgery for rupture.

Answer 128

(a) Gouty tophus in the helix of pinna (ear).

(b) Subchondral bone, olecranon bursa and achilles tendons.

Answer 129

(a) Induration and prominence of soft tissues of the foot.

(b) Pretibial myxoedema.

(c) Graves' disease (thyrotoxicosis).

Answer 130

(a) Peripheral retinal bone corpuscular pigmentation – retinitis pigmentosa.

(b) Night blindness, peripheral visual field constriction and pigmentary retinopathy.

(c) Fifty percent of patients have a family history of the disease inherited in a dominant, recessive or X-linked pattern.

Answer 131

(a) A hazy opacification spreading from the hilar region due to acute left ventricular failure.

(b) Paroxysmal nocturnal dyspnoea, haemoptysis and inspiratory crepitations over the lung bases.

(c) Acute myocardial infarction, hypertension and valvular disease (e.g. aortic stenosis/incompetence).

Answer 132

(a) Cutaneous larva migrans (creeping eruption).

(b) The best-known agents of creeping eruption are the canine hookworms, *Ancylostoma braziliense* and *A. caninum*.

(c) Secondary infection of the lesion.

Answer 133

(a) This shows multiple gouty tophi in the hands.

(b) Aspirated material from the subcutaneous nodule, if examined microscopically, will show typical needle-shaped crystals of monosodium urate monohydrate (gout).

(c) Allopurinol, NSAIDs (e.g. indomethacin), uricosuric drugs (e.g. probenecid) and steroids.

Answer 134

(a) Bradycardia, broad slurred J waves adjacent to the initial QRS deflection, S–T segment depression and T inversion.

(b) Hypothermia.

Answer 135

(a) The bone scan shows increased uptake of the isotope in the left hemipelvis and left femur, in addition to skull vault and bodies of T11 and L1/2/3.

(b) Paget's disease of bone.

Answer 136

(a) Widening of the mediastinum.

(b) Aneurysm of the aorta, lymphadenopathy and other mediastinal tumours, and dissecting aneurysm.

(c) CT scan should be helpful for diagnosis; the individual organs and structures of the mediastinum can be picked out that might be hidden on the simple plain chest radiograph.

Answer 137

(a) Erythema multiforme with lip involvement.
(b) Herpes simplex and mycoplasma.
(c) The lesions may occur over the hands, feet, elbows and knees.

Answer 138

(a) Heavy calcification of the aortic valve.
(b) Severe aortic stenosis.
(c) ECG may show left atrial and ventricular hypertrophy; echocardiography will show an abnormal aortic valve (heavily calcified) and a hypertrophied left ventricle; and doppler cardiography can calculate the systolic gradient across the aortic valve from the velocity of the ejected jet of blood.

Answer 139

(a) This shows stricture at the recto-sigmoid junction with ulceration and polypoid deformity of the mucosa due to carcinoma of the sigmoid colon.
(b) Change of bowel habit (alternate diarrhoea and constipation) and loss of weight.

Answer 140

(a) Gross deformity of hands, and skin atrophy with ecchymosis (and purpura).
(b) Rheumatoid arthritis treated with long-term steroids.

Answer 141

(a) 'Gaucher cell'.
(b) Gaucher's disease (glucocerebrosidosis, glucocerebrosidase deficiency).
(c) Three clinical types: type 1, chronic non-neuronopathic (adult); type 2, acute neuronopathic (infantile); type 3, subacute neuronopathic (juvenile). All types of patients have hepatosplenomegaly and large glucocerebroside-containing reticuloendothelial histiocytes (Gaucher cells) in the marrow.

Answer 142

(a) Erythematous plaques with silvery scales due to psoriasis.
(b) Anywhere – scalp, knees, elbows, thighs, legs, back etc.
(c) Nail involvement and psoriatic arthropathy (which are uncommon in younger patients).

(d) Coal tar preparation, dithranol, topical steroids and ultraviolet radiation may be used for treatment.

Answer 143

(a) This liver biopsy shows, at the centre of the field, a ballooned hepatocyte with clumped eosinophilic hyalin surrounded by rarefied cytoplasm. Note the adjacent neutrophil polymorphs and widespread fatty change.
(b) Alcoholic hepatitis.

Answer 144

(a) (i) This shows calcification in the arch of the aorta showing expansion of the arch, twice the normal due to an aneurysm of the arch of the aorta.
   (ii) It also shows soft tissue shadow in the right paratracheal area which is typical for associated tortuosity of the brachio-cephalic trunk and its branches.
(b) Atherosclerosis (syphilis was once a common cause of ascending aorta aneurysm but has more or less disappeared now).
(c) Pain due to compression on surrounding structures, and aortic valve regurgitation.

Answer 145

(a) Marked wasting of dorsal interossei muscles of the right hand.
(b) Ulnar nerve palsy (may be injured at the elbow).
(c) Injury may occur in those persons who rest their weight on their elbows excessively (occupational), or may occur years following a previously malunited supracondylar fracture of the humerus with bony overgrowth.

Answer 146

(a) Subperiosteal new bone formation in the lower end of tibia.
(b) Hypertrophic pulmonary osteoarthropathy.
(c) (i) Pain in the wrists, ankles, knees and shins
   (ii) Tenderness in the distal parts of long bones of the wrists and ankles
   (iii) Pitting oedema over the anterior aspect of the shin.
(d) X-ray chest for evidence of bronchogenic carcinoma.

Answer 147

(a) The barium enema (lateral radiograph) shows multiple diverticula in a narrowed sigmoid colon.
(b) Lower abdominal pain and disturbed bowel habit (increasing constipation or constipation alternating with diarrhoea).
(c) Rectal bleeding (uncommon but, when it occurs, it tends to be sudden and profuse), diverculitis (pericolitis) and pericolic abscess.

Answer 148

(a) This shows erythema over posterior nail-folds, proximal interphalangeal joints and knuckles due to dermatomyositis.

(b) Muscle weakness involving the proximal limb muscles and anterior neck muscles.

(c) Girls are affected twice as often as boys; the mean age of onset in childhood is about 7 years.

Answer 149

(a) Spidery fingers (arachnodactyly).

(b) Marfan's syndrome.

(c) Phenotypically heterogeneous dominantly inherited.

(d) Skeletal disproportion, i.e. span is greater than height, sternal depression, lens dislocation and a high arched palate.

Answer 150

(a) The X-ray shows calcified lesions of both upper lobes.

(b) Healed pulmonary tuberculosis.

Answer 151

(a) Partial retinal artery occlusion (with a plaque).

(b) Retinal artery occlusion is the result of emboli (atheromatous, myxomatous and material from diseased or artificial heart valves).

(c) Sudden loss of vision.

Answer 152

(a) Narrowing of the joint space and osteophyte formation in the middle and terminal interphalangeal joints, of all the fingers.

(b) Osteoarthritis.

Answer 153

(a) The T-waves are small in all the leads. There is S–T segment depression in I, II, aVF and V4–V6. There are abnormally tall U waves seen in II, aVF and V4–V6 (note that U waves are taller than the preceding T waves); these ECG changes are due to hypokalaemia.

(b) Major causes of hypokalaemia are inadequate intake, excess renal loss (diuretics) and gastrointestinal losses (vomiting and diarrhoea).

(c) Muscle weakness, confusion and paralytic ileus.

Answer 154

(a) Diffuse pulmonary opacities most obvious in the lower zones.

(b) Fibrosing alveolitis.

(c) Progressive exertional breathlessness, clubbing of fingers and numerous bilateral end-inspiratory crepitations (crackles) over the lower zones.

Answer 155

(a) A shiny atrophic plaque of the shin due to necrobiosis lipoidica diabetocorum (minor knocks may precipitate slow-healing ulcers).
(b) Insulin-dependent diabetes mellitus.

Answer 156

(a) *Toxoplasma gondii* in smear of human bone marrow showing half-moon-shaped parasites.
(b) Infection is acquired from the ingestion of cysts excreted in the faeces of infected cats or from eating undercooked beef or lamb.
(c) Toxoplasmosis is a cause of choroidoretinitis and uveitis in adults.

Answer 157

(a) Typical bamboo spine due to ankylosing spondylitis.
(b) Recurring episodes of low back pain aggravated by breathing resulting from involvement of the costovertebral joints and failure to obliterate the lumbar lordosis on forward flexion.
(c) Iritis, aortic regurgitation, apical pulmonary fibrosis and osteoporosis.

Answer 158

(a) Inflammatory skin nodules (discrete at first but some becoming confluent) due to erythema nodosum. Note also associated ankle swelling.
(b) Streptococcal infection and primary tuberculous infection.

Answer 159

(a) The CT scan shows right pleural effusion, the characteristic features are the shape and its density between muscle and fat.
(b) Pneumonia, pulmonary infarction, malignant disease and tuberculosis.

Answer 160

(a) This shows a soft tissue mass based on the mediastinum extending into the right and left lung fields due to lymphadenopathy.
(b) Lymphoma, Hodgkin's disease and secondary from carcinoma of bronchus.

Index of cases by question number